THE POWER OF BETA GLUCAN:

HOW DIETARY FIBER CAN COMBAT OBESITY AND METABOLIC SYNDROMES

Xu-Feng Huang, MD, PhD, DSc

Professor of Medical Science

School of Medical, Indigenous, and Health Sciences
The University of Wollongong
Australia
2023

Ashahi-Maple

National Library of Australia Cataloguing-in-Publication Data is available.

First published in Australia in 2023
by Ashahi-Maple©, Inc.

ISBN 978-0-6454760-4-0

TO MY FAMILY

Preface

This book is for anyone interested in improving their health, especially those struggling with obesity, metabolic syndromes, and related conditions.

It aims to provide a comprehensive understanding of dietary fiber, specifically beta-glucan, its benefits, and how to incorporate it into the diet. The book offers practical tips, resources, and delicious recipes to help readers achieve their health goals. Additionally, it discusses the causes and consequences of obesity and metabolic syndromes, and provides insights on who should avoid high fiber diets.

Overall, the book educates readers about the benefits of beta-glucan in promoting a healthy lifestyle and combating health-related issues.

Professor Xu-Feng Huang, MD, PhD, DSc

CONTENTS

CHAPTER 1: OBESITY AND METABOLIC SYNDROME

OBESITY

Overweight and obesity

Being overweight and obese are conditions characterized by excessive accumulation of body fat that can adversely affect health.

Being overweight or obese can increase the risk of many health problems, including type 2 diabetes, high blood pressure, heart disease, stroke, sleep apnea, and certain types of cancer. These conditions can significantly reduce the quality of life and may even be life-threatening.

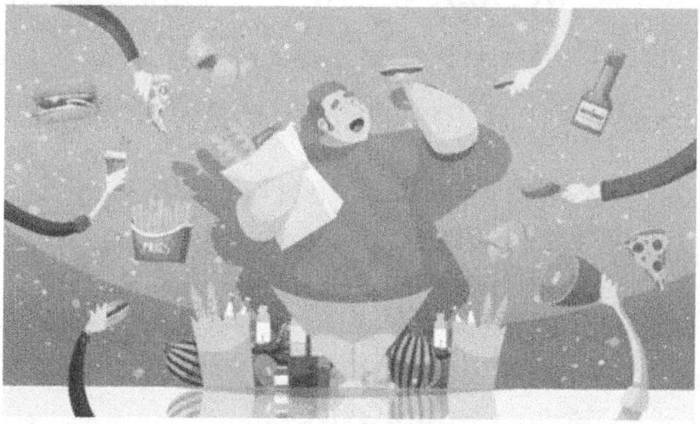

The primary causes of overweight and obesity are an imbalance between energy intake (calories consumed) and energy expenditure (calories burned through physical activity and bodily processes). Factors contributing to this imbalance include a poor diet, lack of physical activity, genetic predisposition, and certain medical conditions and medications.

Treatment of overweight and obesity typically involves lifestyle modifications, such as increasing physical activity and improving dietary habits. Medications or surgical interventions may sometimes be recommended to help manage the condition. Working with a healthcare professional to determine the best approach for an individual's specific needs is important.

Obesity and body mass index

Body mass index (BMI) is a commonly used tool to assess whether an individual's weight falls within a healthy range for their height. BMI is calculated by dividing a person's weight in kilograms by their height in meters squared.

1. Normal weight: BMI between 18.5 and 24.9
2. Overweight: BMI between 25.0 and 29.9
3. Obese: BMI between 30.0 and 34.9 (Class I), BMI between 35.0 and 39.9 (Class II)
4. Severe obese: BMI of 40 or higher (Class III)

However, it's important to note that BMI is not a perfect measure of body fat. Other factors such as muscle mass, age, and ethnicity may affect the interpretation of BMI results.

It's important to note that while BMI can be a valuable tool for assessing weight status and health risks, it should not be used as the sole health measure. Other factors, such as blood pressure, cholesterol, and blood sugar levels, may also need to be considered. It's always best to talk with a healthcare professional about your health risks and how to manage them.

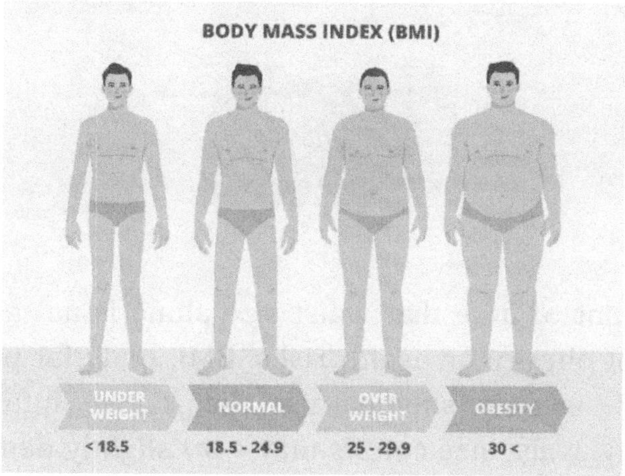

Therefore, healthcare providers may use a combination of BMI, waist circumference, and other health markers to assess an individual's overall health and risk of health problems related to weight.

Waist size of obesity

Waist size can be an indicator of obesity and increased health risks. Generally, a waist circumference greater than 102 cm (40 inches) for men and greater than 88 cm (35 inches) for women is considered a risk factor for metabolic syndrome and other health problems associated with obesity. This is because excess abdominal fat can be a sign of increased visceral fat, which surrounds the organs in the abdomen and can contribute to inflammation and insulin resistance.

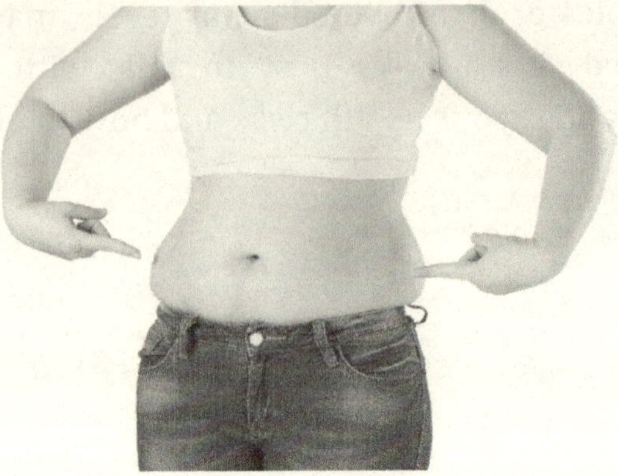

It's important to note that waist size alone is not a definitive indicator of obesity or health risks. BMI, body fat percentage, and other factors should also be taken into account. Additionally, waist size cutoffs may vary slightly depending on the population being studied or the specific health outcomes of interest.

Causes of overweight and obesity

Overweight and obesity are caused by an imbalance between energy intake (calories consumed) and energy expenditure (calories burned through physical activity and bodily processes). This means consuming more calories than the body burns leads to excess body fat storage, leading to obesity.

The following are some common factors that can contribute to this energy imbalance:

1. Poor dietary habits: Consuming large amounts of calorie-dense, nutrient-poor foods such as fast food, sugary drinks, and snacks can contribute to weight gain.

2. Lack of physical activity: Sedentary lifestyles can lead to a decrease in energy expenditure, such as sitting for long periods at work or at home, and not engaging in regular exercise,
3. Genetics: Certain genetic factors can make it more difficult for some people to lose weight or regulate their appetite.
4. Medical conditions: Certain conditions, such as hypothyroidism, Cushing's syndrome, and polycystic ovary syndrome (PCOS), can contribute to weight gain.
5. Medications: Certain medications, such as antidepressants, antipsychotics, and corticosteroids, can cause weight gain as a side effect.
6. Psychological factors: Emotional eating, stress, and lack of sleep can contribute to overeating and weight gain.

It's important to note that being overweight and obesity are complex conditions, and multiple factors may be at play. However, addressing these factors through lifestyle modifications and seeking support from a healthcare professional can help manage and prevent weight gain.

Consequences of obesity

Obesity can lead to several negative health consequences, including:

1. Type 2 diabetes: Obesity is a significant risk factor for developing type 2 diabetes. Excess body fat can interfere with the body's ability to use insulin to regulate blood sugar levels properly.

2. Cardiovascular disease: Excess body fat can contribute to high blood pressure, high cholesterol, and inflammation, all of which can increase the risk of heart disease, stroke, and other cardiovascular problems.
3. Respiratory problems: Obesity can lead to breathing difficulties, such as sleep apnea, asthma, and shortness of breath.
4. Joint problems: The excess weight can put extra stress on joints, which can lead to conditions such as osteoarthritis.
5. Increased risk of certain cancers: Obesity has been linked to an increased risk of several types of cancer, including breast, colon, and pancreatic cancer.
6. Mental health problems: Obesity has been associated with depression, anxiety, and other mental health issues.

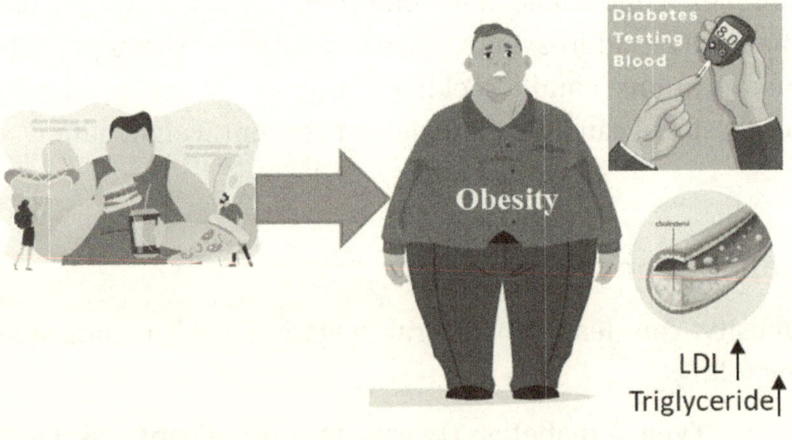

Management of obesity

The management of obesity involves making changes to both dietary and lifestyle habits. Here are some strategies that can help manage obesity:

1. Dietary changes: Reducing calorie intake by choosing healthier foods and reducing portion sizes can effectively manage obesity. A diet rich in fruits, vegetables, whole grains, lean proteins, and healthy fats can help promote weight loss.
2. Physical activity: Regular physical activity is essential for weight management and overall health. Aim for at least 120 minutes of moderate-intensity weekly exercise, such as brisk walking.
3. Behavior modification: Changing habits and behaviors related to food and physical activity can help promote long-term weight management. Setting realistic goals, monitoring progress, and seeking support from a healthcare professional can help achieve success.
4. Medications: Certain medications can be prescribed to help manage obesity, such as appetite suppressants and medications that interfere with fat absorption.

It's important to note that weight management is a long-term process, and success often requires a combination of these strategies. Seeking support from healthcare professionals, such as a registered dietitian, a personal trainer, or a physician, can help identify the most effective methods for individual needs and goals.

METABOLIC SYNDROME

Definition

Metabolic syndrome is a cluster of conditions that often occur together and increase the risk of developing cardiovascular disease, type 2 diabetes, and other health problems. These risk factors include:

1. Abdominal obesity: Excessive fat around the waist.
2. High blood pressure: Blood pressure levels of 130/85 mmHg or higher.
3. High blood sugar levels: Fasting blood sugar levels of 5.6 mmol/L or higher.
4. Elevated triglycerides: Triglyceride levels of 1.7 mmol/L or higher.
5. Low levels of HDL cholesterol: HDL cholesterol levels below 1.03 mmol/L for men and 1.30 mmol/L for women.

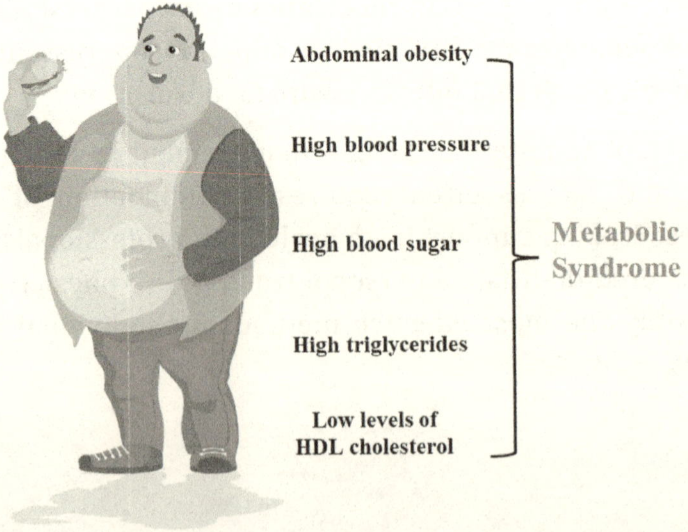

Causes of metabolic syndrome

Causes of obesity and metabolic syndrome are complex conditions that arise from genetic, environmental, and lifestyle factors. Some of the leading causes and contributing factors to obesity and metabolic syndrome include:

1. Unhealthy diet: A diet high in calories, saturated and trans fats, sugar, and processed foods can contribute to obesity and metabolic syndrome.
2. Lack of physical activity: A sedentary lifestyle and lack of regular exercise can contribute to obesity and metabolic abnormalities.

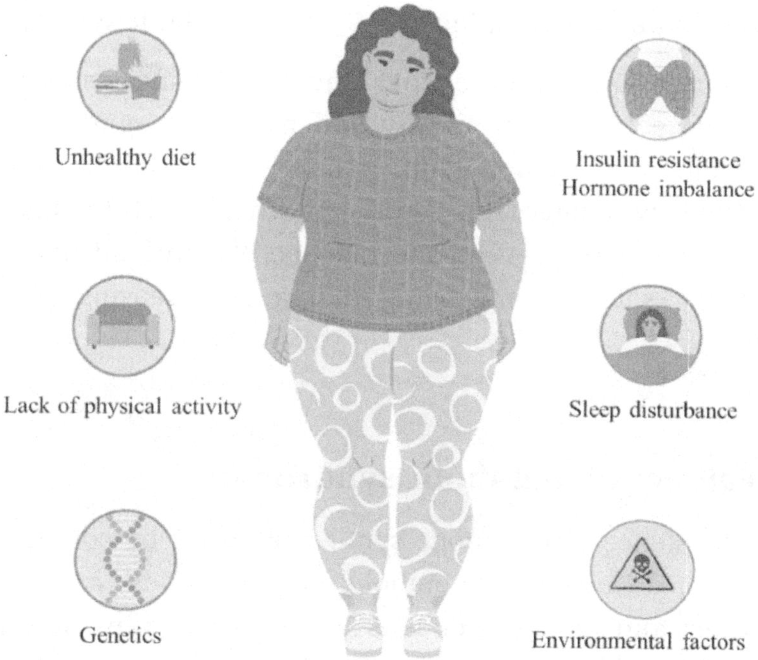

3. Genetics: Certain genetic factors may make some individuals more prone to developing obesity and metabolic syndrome.

4. Insulin resistance: Insulin resistance, a condition in which the body's cells become less responsive to insulin, can contribute to high blood sugar levels, type 2 diabetes, and metabolic syndrome.

5. Hormonal imbalances: Certain hormonal imbalances, such as those related to thyroid function or menopause, may contribute to the development of obesity and metabolic syndrome.

6. Sleep disturbances: Lack of sleep and sleep disorders, such as sleep apnea, have been linked to an increased risk of obesity and metabolic syndrome.

7. Environmental factors: Environmental factors, such as exposure to certain chemicals, toxins, and pollutants, may contribute to developing obesity and metabolic syndrome.

It is important to note that the underlying causes and contributing factors to obesity and metabolic syndrome can vary from person to person, and not everyone with these conditions will have the same underlying factors. Lifestyle changes can help prevent and manage obesity and metabolic syndrome, such as improving diet and increasing physical activity.

Prevalence of metabolic syndrome

The prevalence of metabolic syndrome varies by country and population. However, metabolic syndrome is a common condition, and its prevalence is increasing worldwide due to rising rates of obesity, physical inactivity, and unhealthy dietary habits. Early detection and management of metabolic syndrome can help prevent or delay the development of cardiovascular disease and type 2 diabetes.

Complications of metabolic syndrome

Metabolic syndrome is a cluster of metabolic disorders that increase the risk of cardiovascular disease, type 2 diabetes, and other health problems.

Some of the complications that can arise from metabolic syndrome include:

1. Cardiovascular disease: People with metabolic syndrome are at an increased risk of developing cardiovascular disease, including heart attack and stroke. This is because the syndrome can cause atherosclerosis, a plaque buildup in the arteries that can narrow and harden them.
2. Type 2 diabetes: Metabolic syndrome is strongly associated with insulin resistance, a condition in which the body's cells become less responsive to insulin. This can lead to high blood sugar levels and type 2 diabetes.
3. Kidney disease: Metabolic syndrome can damage the kidneys and increase the risk of chronic kidney disease and kidney failure.
4. Non-alcoholic fatty liver disease: Metabolic syndrome can lead to the accumulation of fat in the liver, which can cause inflammation and damage to liver cells.
5. Sleep apnea: Metabolic syndrome is associated with sleep apnea, a condition in which a person's breathing is repeatedly interrupted during sleep.
6. Polycystic ovary syndrome (PCOS): Metabolic syndrome is also associated with PCOS, a hormonal disorder that

can cause irregular periods, infertility, and other health problems in women.

7. Cancer: Some studies have suggested that metabolic syndrome may increase the risk of certain types of cancer, including breast and colon cancer.

Overall, metabolic syndrome can have serious health consequences if left untreated, making it important to manage the underlying risk factors through lifestyle changes and medical interventions.

Management of metabolic syndrome

Management of metabolic syndrome involves making lifestyle changes and receiving medical treatment as needed. Here are some steps that can be taken to manage metabolic syndrome:

1. Eat a healthy diet: Eating a diet that is low in saturated and trans fats, added sugars, and sodium can help improve metabolic parameters. Focus on a diet that is rich in vegetables, fruits, whole grains, lean protein, and healthy fats.
2. Exercise regularly: Regular physical activity can help improve insulin sensitivity, blood pressure, and lipid profiles. Aim for at least 150 minutes of moderate-intensity or 75 minutes of vigorous weekly exercise.
3. Lose weight: Losing weight, especially abdominal fat, can help improve metabolic parameters. As a result, even modest weight loss can significantly reduce the risk of cardiovascular disease and type 2 diabetes.
4. Manage stress: Chronic stress can contribute to insulin resistance and inflammation, so finding ways to manage

stress, such as meditation or relaxation techniques, can be helpful.

5. Quit smoking: Smoking can worsen insulin resistance and increase the risk of cardiovascular disease, so quitting smoking is an essential step in managing metabolic syndrome.
6. Medications: Depending on individual circumstances, medications may be prescribed to help control blood pressure, cholesterol, and blood sugar levels.
7. Regular monitoring: Regular check-ups with a healthcare provider can help track progress and ensure that any necessary adjustments are made to the management plan.

Overall, managing metabolic syndrome is focused on reducing risk factors through lifestyle changes and, if necessary, medication. With proper management, it is possible to improve metabolic parameters and reduce the risk of complications associated with metabolic syndrome.

CHAPTER 2: DIETARY FIBER AND BETA-GLUCAN

DIETARY FIBER

What is dietary fiber?

Dietary fiber refers to the indigestible components of plant foods that pass relatively intact through the digestive system. It includes complex carbohydrates, such as cellulose, hemicellulose, and pectin, that are found in fruits, vegetables, whole grains, nuts, and seeds. Unlike other nutrients, such as proteins, fats, and carbohydrates, dietary fiber is not digested or absorbed by the body. Instead, it passes through the digestive tract essentially unchanged, helping to regulate digestion and prevent constipation.

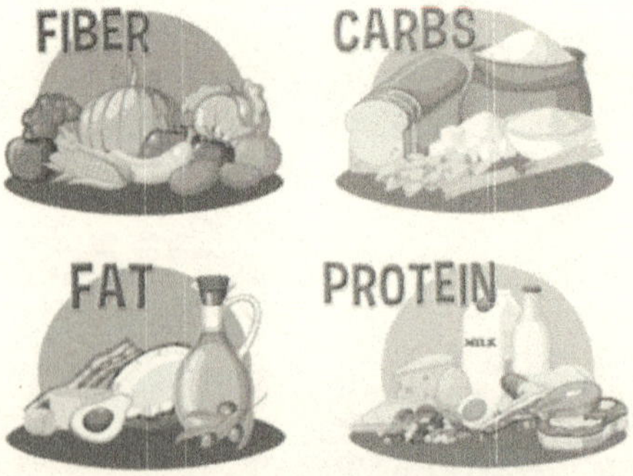

The trend of global dietary fiber intake

The trend of dietary fiber intake over the last 70 years in many countries has been a significant decrease. This is due to the increasing consumption of processed foods and a reduction in the consumption of whole foods, such as fruits, vegetables, and whole grains, which are rich sources of dietary fiber.

For example, in the United States, the average daily fiber intake for adults is around 15 grams, which is well below the recommended intake of 25 grams for women and 38 grams for men. In the 1950s, the average daily fiber intake in the US was around 20-25 grams, which was closer to the recommended intake. However, with the rise of processed foods and a decrease in the consumption of whole foods, fiber intake has steadily decreased over the decades.

A similar trend has been observed in countries such as the UK, Canada, and Australia, where the average fiber intake has decreased over time. The decline in fiber intake is a concern as it has been linked to an increased risk of chronic diseases such as obesity, type 2 diabetes, and cardiovascular disease.

To address this issue, various public health campaigns and initiatives have been implemented to increase awareness of the importance of dietary fiber and encourage individuals to consume more fiber-rich foods. These efforts aim to reverse the trend of declining fiber intake and promote better health outcomes.

Fiber intake and chronic diseases

The trend of decreasing dietary fiber intake over the last 70 years is associated with an increased risk of several chronic diseases. This is because dietary fiber plays an essential role in maintaining gut health, regulating blood sugar levels, and reducing inflammation, all of which are important for preventing chronic diseases.

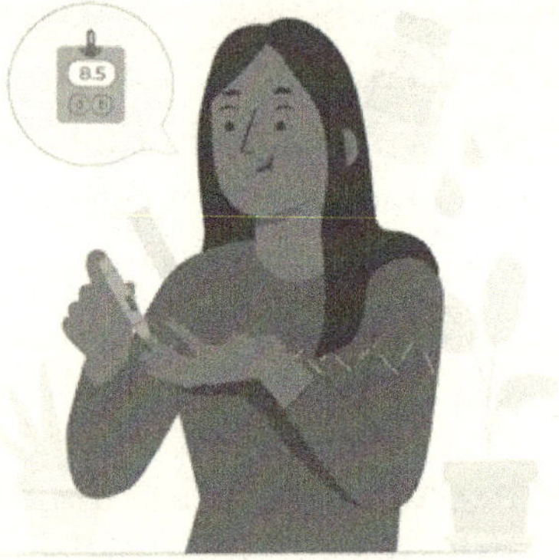

One of the main risks associated with low fiber intake is an increased risk of developing obesity. Fiber helps to increase satiety and reduce energy intake, which can help to prevent overeating and weight gain. Low fiber intake has also been linked to an increased risk of type 2 diabetes, as fiber can help to regulate blood sugar levels and improve insulin sensitivity.

In addition, low fiber intake has been linked to an increased risk of cardiovascular disease, as fiber can help to reduce LDL (bad) cholesterol levels and improve heart health. Low fiber intake has also been associated with an increased risk of certain types of cancer, particularly colorectal cancer, as fiber can help promote gut health and reduce inflammation.

Types of dietary fiber

There are two main types of dietary fiber: soluble fiber and insoluble fiber.

1. Soluble fiber: This type of fiber dissolves in water and forms a gel-like substance in the digestive tract. Soluble fiber is found in oats, barley, psyllium, beans, peas, lentils, apples, oranges, and carrots. It has been shown to help lower cholesterol levels, regulate blood sugar levels, and promote a feeling of fullness.

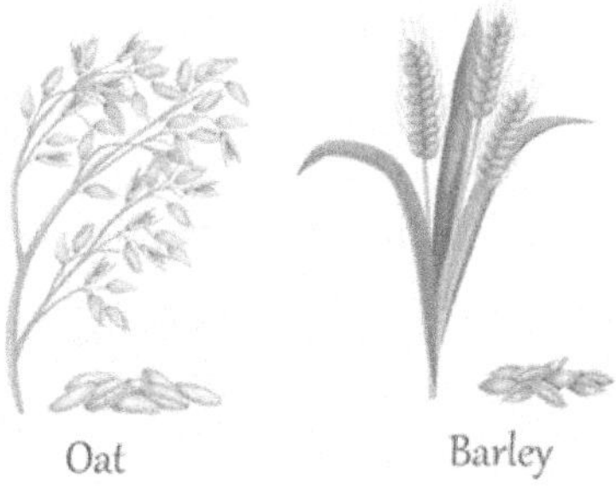

2. Insoluble fiber: This type of fiber does not dissolve in water and helps to move food through the digestive system. Insoluble fiber is found in whole grains, nuts, seeds, fruits, and vegetables. It helps to promote regular bowel movements and prevent constipation.

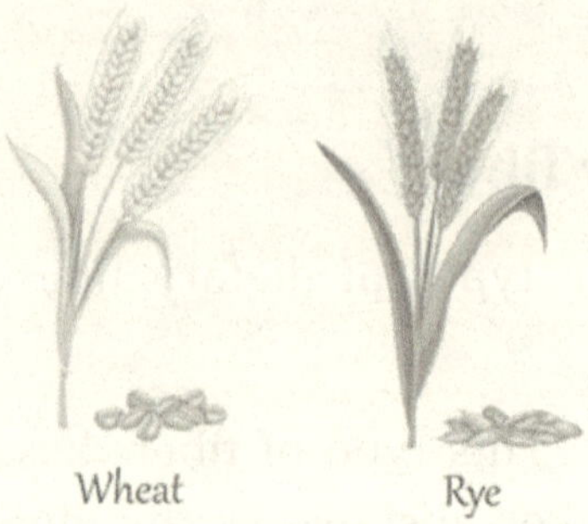

Both types of fiber are essential for maintaining good health and preventing chronic diseases, such as heart disease, diabetes, and certain types of cancer. It is recommended that adults consume 25-30 grams of fiber per day from a variety of food sources.

Soluble fiber

Soluble fiber is a type of dietary fiber that dissolves in water to form a gel-like substance in the digestive tract. Here are some of its essential characteristics, sources, health benefits, and potential side effects:

Compositions: Soluble fiber is composed of complex carbohydrates, such as pectins, gums, and beta-glucans, that are found in plant-based foods.

Characteristics: Soluble fiber absorbs water and swells in the digestive tract, which can help to slow down the absorption of nutrients, regulate blood sugar levels, and promote feelings of fullness. It can also bind to cholesterol in the digestive tract and help to lower blood cholesterol levels.

Sources: Soluble fiber is found in various plant-based foods, including oats, barley, psyllium, beans, peas, lentils, apples, oranges, strawberries, blueberries, carrots, and sweet potatoes.

Health benefits: Consuming soluble fiber can have several health benefits, including:

- Lowering cholesterol levels: Soluble fiber can bind to cholesterol in the digestive tract and help lower blood cholesterol levels, reducing the risk of heart disease.
- Regulating blood sugar levels: Soluble fiber can slow down the absorption of carbohydrates in the digestive tract, which can help to regulate blood sugar levels and reduce the risk of diabetes.
- Promoting feelings of fullness: Soluble fiber can help to promote feelings of fullness and reduce the risk of overeating and weight gain.
- Improving gut health: Soluble fiber can help feed the beneficial bacteria in the gut, improving gut health and reducing the risk of digestive disorders.

Side effects: Consuming too much soluble fiber can cause bloating, gas, and diarrhea in some people, especially if they are not used to high-fiber foods. It is important to gradually increase fiber intake over time and drink plenty of water to avoid these side effects.

Foods from the highest to lowest soluble fibers

Here are some examples of foods ranked from highest to lowest in terms of their soluble fiber content per serving:

1. Oats: Oat bran and rolled oats are high in soluble fiber, with around 1-2 grams of soluble fiber per half-cup serving.
2. Legumes: Lentils, peas, and beans (such as black beans, kidney beans, navy beans, and lima beans) are excellent

sources of soluble fiber, with around 1-2 grams of soluble fiber per half-cup serving.

3. Nuts and Seeds: Chia seeds, flaxseeds, and sunflower seeds are good sources of soluble fiber, with around 1 gram of soluble fiber per tablespoon serving.

4. Fruits: Some fruits are also high in soluble fiber, including apples, pears, bananas, and berries. One medium-sized apple contains around 1 gram of soluble fiber.

5. Vegetables: Vegetables such as Brussels sprouts, sweet potatoes, and broccoli are also good sources of soluble fiber, with around 1-2 grams of soluble fiber per half-cup serving.

It's important to note that the exact amount of soluble fiber in foods can vary depending on the type of food, how it is prepared, and the serving size. Nonetheless, including various high-fiber foods in your diet can help you meet your daily fiber needs and support good digestive health.

Insoluble fiber

Insoluble fiber is an essential component of a healthy diet. Here are some key characteristics, sources, health benefits, and side effects of insoluble fiber:

Compositions: Insoluble fiber is composed of plant cell walls that the digestive system cannot break down. These cell walls include cellulose, hemicellulose, and lignin.

Characteristics: Insoluble fiber is not soluble in water and is not broken down by the digestive system. Instead, it helps to move food through the digestive tract by adding bulk and promoting regular bowel movements. Because the body does not break down insoluble fiber, it provides no calories.

Sources: Insoluble fiber is found in many plant-based foods, including:

- Whole grains: wheat, oats, barley, quinoa, brown rice, and bulgur
- Nuts and seeds: almonds, pecans, walnuts, sunflower seeds, and sesame seeds
- Fruits and vegetables: broccoli, carrots, cauliflower, green beans, apples, and berries

Health benefits: Insoluble fiber has several health benefits, including:

- Promoting regular bowel movements: Insoluble fiber adds bulk to stool, which helps to promote regular bowel movements and prevent constipation.
- Reducing the risk of colon cancer: Insoluble fiber helps to move food through the digestive system more quickly, which reduces the amount of time that potentially harmful substances stay in contact with the colon lining.
- Improving satiety: Insoluble fiber adds bulk to food, which can help you feel full for longer and reduce your overall calorie intake.

Side effects: Consuming too much insoluble fiber can cause some side effects, including:

- Bloating and gas: Insoluble fiber can ferment in the colon, which can cause gas and bloating.
- Diarrhea: Consuming large amounts of insoluble fiber without drinking enough water can cause diarrhea.

- Dehydration: Insoluble fiber absorbs water as it moves through the digestive system, so drinking plenty of water is important to prevent dehydration.

Dietary fiber intake and obesity

There is a well-established relationship between dietary fiber intake and obesity. Numerous studies have shown that people who consume higher amounts of dietary fiber tend to have a lower risk of obesity.

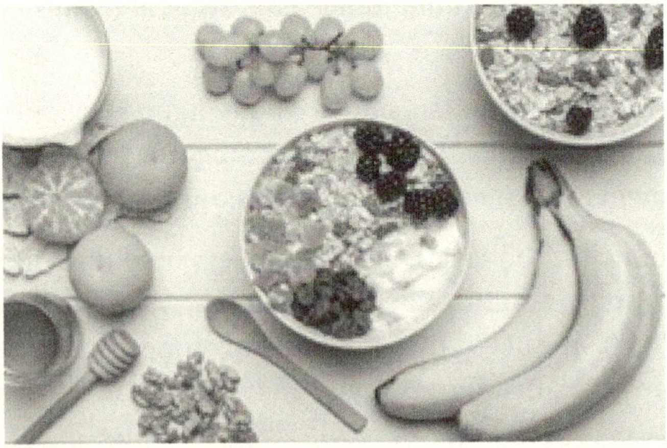

One of the main reasons for this is that dietary fiber helps to promote feelings of fullness and satiety, which can reduce overall calorie intake. Fiber also slows down the absorption of carbohydrates, which can help regulate blood sugar levels and prevent overeating.

Furthermore, foods high in fiber, such as fruits, vegetables, whole grains, and legumes, tend to be lower in calories and nutrients than processed and high-fat foods. Therefore, by replacing high-calorie, low-nutrient foods with fiber-rich foods, individuals may be able to reduce their calorie intake and maintain a healthy weight.

Research also suggests that certain fiber types, such as soluble fiber, may be particularly beneficial for weight management. Soluble fiber forms a gel-like substance in the digestive tract, which can help slow down the absorption of nutrients and regulate appetite.

Increasing dietary fiber intake is a healthy and effective way to promote weight loss and prevent obesity. However, it is important to note that simply increasing fiber intake alone may not be enough to achieve significant weight loss. A healthy and balanced diet and regular exercise are essential for maintaining a healthy weight.

Dietary fiber and metabolic syndrome

Studies have shown a strong relationship between dietary fiber intake and metabolic syndrome.

The relationship between dietary fiber intake and metabolic syndrome is clear (Pal et al., 2011). Therefore, consuming a diet high in fiber-rich foods can help to prevent the development of the metabolic syndrome and improve the symptoms of those who already have it.

Foods rich in insoluble fibers

Here is a list of foods that are high in insoluble fiber, ranked from highest to lowest:

1. Bran cereal (1 cup): 22.3 grams of insoluble fiber

2. Whole wheat flour (1 cup): 13.2 grams of insoluble fiber
3. Wheat bran (1 cup): 12.8 grams of insoluble fiber
4. Popcorn (1 cup popped): 1.2 grams of insoluble fiber
5. Brown rice (1 cup cooked): 1.2 grams of insoluble fiber
6. Almonds (1 ounce): 3.5 grams of insoluble fiber
7. Pistachios (1 ounce): 2.8 grams of insoluble fiber
8. Carrots (1 cup chopped): 3.4 grams of insoluble fiber
9. Broccoli (1 cup chopped): 2.6 grams of insoluble fiber
10. Sweet potato (1 medium): 3.8 grams of insoluble fiber

It's worth noting that many high-fiber foods contain soluble and insoluble fiber, and the amount of fiber in a food can vary depending on how it's prepared. So eating a variety of whole, plant-based foods is the best way to ensure you get enough fiber.

How much dietary fiber do we need per day?

The recommended daily fiber intake for adults is 25-30 grams per day, which should include a mix of soluble and insoluble fiber. While there is no specific daily requirement for soluble fiber, most health experts recommend balancing both fiber types for optimal health benefits.

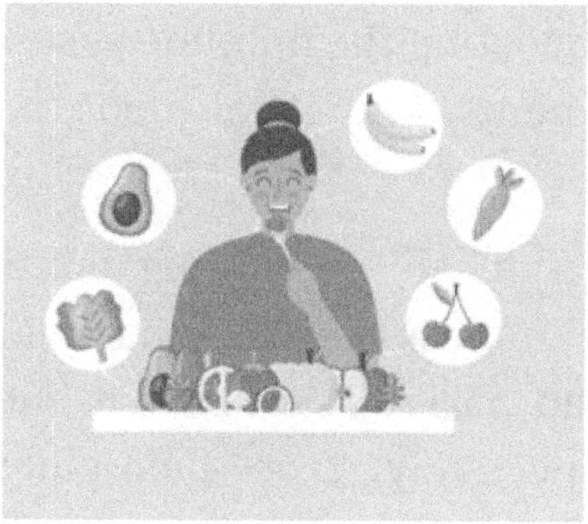

According to the Institute of Medicine, the recommended soluble fiber intake is 10-15 grams daily. However, individual needs may vary based on factors such as age, sex, and activity level.

Consuming enough soluble fiber can help lower cholesterol levels, regulate blood sugar levels, and promote a feeling of fullness, supporting healthy weight management. To increase your soluble fiber intake, you can include sources such as legumes, oats, nuts and seeds, fruits, and vegetables.

As always, it's essential to talk to your doctor or a registered dietitian before making any significant changes to your diet, especially if you have any underlying health conditions or dietary restrictions.

BETA-GLUCAN

Beta-glucan is a type of soluble fiber that is found in various sources, such as oats, barley, yeast, and certain types of mushrooms. It is a complex polysaccharide made up of chains of glucose molecules that are linked together in a particular way.

Beta-glucan is known for its various health benefits, such as improving heart health by reducing cholesterol levels, regulating blood sugar levels, and boosting the immune system. It is often used in dietary supplements, functional foods, and cosmetics.

There are different types of beta-glucan, depending on the source and the way the glucose molecules are linked. For example, beta-glucan from oats and barley is called oat beta-glucan or barley beta-glucan, respectively. Yeast beta-glucan and mushroom beta-glucan are also common sources of this fiber.

Type of beta-glucan by sources

Beta-glucans are a group of polysaccharides (complex carbohydrates) found in various organisms' cell walls, including bacteria, fungi, yeasts, algae, and plants. They are known for their health benefits, including their immune-stimulating and cholesterol-lowering properties.

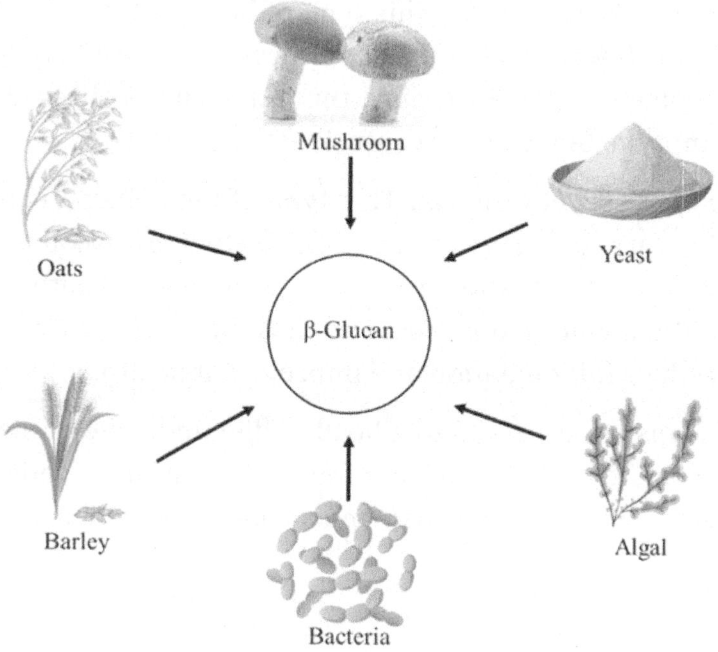

There are several types of beta-glucans, including:

1. Yeast Beta-Glucan: This type of beta-glucan is extracted from the cell walls of baker's yeast (Saccharomyces cerevisiae). It is commonly used as a dietary supplement to support the immune system and reduce the risk of infections.

2. Mushroom Beta-Glucan: This type of beta-glucan is found in the cell walls of various mushroom species, including shiitake, maitake, and reishi mushrooms. It is known for its immune-stimulating properties and has been shown to help reduce inflammation and fight cancer.

3. Oat Beta-Glucan: This type of beta-glucan is found in the soluble fiber of oats. It has been shown to help reduce LDL ("bad") cholesterol levels, lower blood sugar levels and improve digestive health.

4. Barley Beta-Glucan: This type of beta-glucan is found in the cell walls of barley. It has been shown to help lower cholesterol levels, reduce the risk of heart disease, and improve blood sugar control.
5. Seaweed Beta-Glucan: This type of beta-glucan is found in various seaweed species, including wakame and kombu. It is known for its immune-stimulating and antioxidant properties and has been shown to help reduce inflammation and improve gut health.

Beta-glucans are essential to a healthy diet and have numerous health benefits. They can be found in various foods and supplements, including yeast, mushrooms, oats, barley, and seaweed.

Types of beta-glucan by chemical structures

Beta-glucans are a diverse group of complex polysaccharides characterized by their β-(1,3)-D-glucan backbone and β-(1,6)-D-glucan side chains. There are different types of beta-glucans, which can be classified based on their chemical structures. Here are some examples:

1. Linear beta-glucans: These are the simplest type of beta-glucans, composed only of β-(1,3)-D-glucose residues without side chains.
2. Branched beta-glucans: These beta-glucans have β-(1,6)-D-glucose side chains attached to the β-(1,3)-D-glucose backbone.
3. Mixed-linkage beta-glucans: These beta-glucans have both β-(1,3)-D-glucose and β-(1,4)-D-glucose linkages, in addition to β-(1,6)-D-glucose side chains.

4. Fungal beta-glucans: These beta-glucans are commonly found in fungi and have a complex structure with β-(1,3)-D-glucose and β-(1,6)-D-glucose linkages in the main chain, and β-(1,3)-D-glucose, β-(1,6)-D-glucose, and β-(1,4)-D-glucose linkages in the side chains.
5. Cereal beta-glucans: These beta-glucans are found in the endosperm cell walls of cereal grains and have a mixed-linkage structure with β-(1,3)-D-glucose and β-(1,4)-D-glucose linkages in the main chain and β-(1,3)-D-glucose side chains.
6. Yeast beta-glucans: These beta-glucans are commonly found in yeast cell walls and have a linear structure with β-(1,3)-D-glucose linkages.

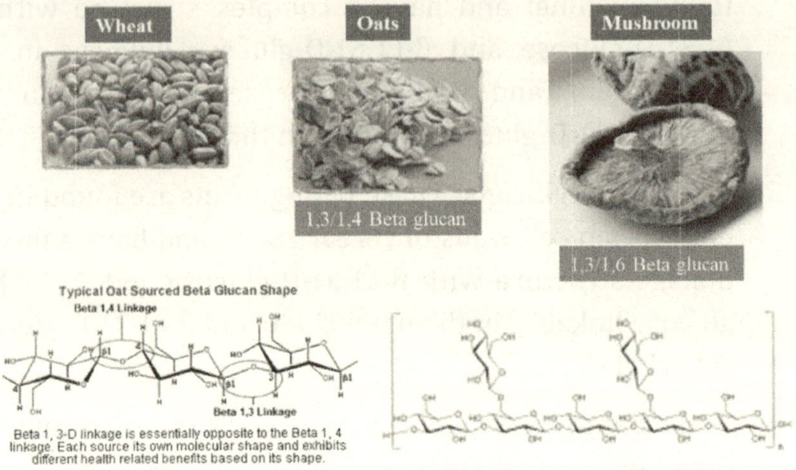

These are just some examples of the different types of beta-glucans that exist. The chemical structure of beta-glucans can vary depending on the source from which they are derived.

Slow down absorption

When beta-glucan is consumed, it forms a gel-like substance in the digestive tract, similar to other types of soluble fiber. This gel-like substance slows down glucose absorption into the bloodstream, helping regulate blood sugar levels.

Beta-glucan also binds to bile acids in the digestive tract, which are necessary for the digestion and absorption of fat. This binding process reduces the amount of bile acids available for fat digestion, which can decrease cholesterol levels.

Immune-boosting beta-glucans

It's important to note that the strength of immune-boosting effects can vary depending on factors such as the dose, purity, and form of beta-glucan used and an individual's overall health status. That being said, here are some beta-glucans that have been shown to have immune-boosting effects, starting from the strongest based on available research:

1. Beta-glucans from certain strains of mushrooms: Beta-glucans derived from certain types of mushrooms, such as shiitake, maitake, and reishi, have been extensively studied for their immune-boosting properties. These beta-glucans have been shown to activate various immune cells, including macrophages and natural killer cells, and may also have anti-inflammatory effects.

2. Beta-glucans from yeast: Beta-glucans derived from baker's yeast, specifically beta-1,3/1,6-glucan, have been shown to enhance immune function. This type of beta-glucan has been found to activate macrophages and other immune cells and may also help stimulate antibody production.

3. Oat beta-glucan: Oat beta-glucan has been studied for its immune-boosting properties, particularly its ability to enhance the activity of white blood cells known as neutrophils.

4. Seaweed beta-glucans: Some studies suggest that certain types of seaweed-derived beta-glucans, such as those found in brown seaweed, may have immune-boosting effects. These beta-glucans have been shown to activate immune cells and may also have antioxidant and anti-inflammatory effects.

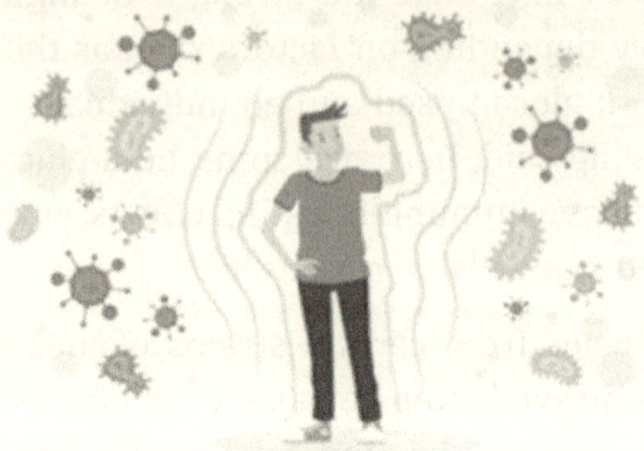

It's important to note that while beta-glucans can benefit immune function, they should not be relied upon as a sole treatment for any health condition. As always, talking to a healthcare provider before starting any new supplement or making significant changes to your diet or lifestyle is important.

The molecular mechanisms on health

The molecular mechanism by which beta-glucans exert their effects on health is complex and involves several pathways in the body. Here are some of the key mechanisms by which beta-glucans may impact health:

1. Immune modulation: Beta-glucans have been shown to stimulate immune cells, including macrophages, natural killer cells, and neutrophils, which play a key role in defending the body against infection and disease. This activation of immune cells is thought to occur through the binding of beta-glucans to specific receptors on the surface of immune cells, which triggers a series of signaling pathways that lead to immune activation.

2. Anti-inflammatory effects: Beta-glucans may also have anti-inflammatory effects by modulating the activity of inflammatory molecules in the body. This can help reduce inflammation, which is thought to play a role in developing chronic diseases such as heart disease, diabetes, and cancer.
3. Cholesterol-lowering effects: Certain beta-glucans, such as those found in oats and barley, have been shown to reduce cholesterol levels by binding to bile acids in the gut and reducing their reabsorption. This leads to an increase in the excretion of bile acids, which reduces the amount of cholesterol produced by the liver.
4. Blood sugar regulation: Beta-glucans may also help regulate blood sugar levels by slowing down the absorption of carbohydrates in the gut and reducing insulin resistance. This can help prevent spikes in blood sugar levels, which can lead to diabetes and other metabolic disorders.

Beta-glucan supplements

Many different beta-glucan supplements are available on the market, making it difficult to know which one to choose. However, here are some of the most common types of beta-glucan supplements, along with their daily doses:

1. Mushroom beta-glucans: Mushroom-derived beta-glucans are one of the most common beta-glucan supplements on the market. These supplements typically contain beta-glucans derived from shiitake, maitake, or reishi mushrooms and are often marketed for their immune-boosting effects. Daily doses of

mushroom beta-glucan supplements can vary but typically range from 100 to 500 mg daily.

2. Yeast beta-glucans: Yeast-derived beta-glucans are another common type of beta-glucan supplement. These supplements typically contain beta-1,3/1,6-glucan, which has been shown to have immune-boosting effects. Daily doses of yeast beta-glucan supplements can vary but typically range from 100 to 500 mg daily.

3. Oat beta-glucans: Oat beta-glucans are a type of soluble fiber that has been shown to have cholesterol-lowering effects. Oat beta-glucan supplements typically contain concentrated oat beta-glucans and may be marketed for their cholesterol-lowering or blood sugar-regulating effects. Daily doses of oat beta-glucan supplements usually range from 3 to 5 grams.

4. Barley beta-glucans: Barley beta-glucans are another type of soluble fiber that has been shown to have cholesterol-lowering effects. Barley beta-glucan supplements typically contain concentrated forms of barley beta-glucans and may be marketed for their cholesterol-lowering or blood sugar-regulating effects. Daily doses of barley beta-glucan supplements usually range from 3 to 5 grams.

When choosing a beta-glucan supplement, it's essential to look for a product tested for purity and potency and follow the manufacturer's recommended dosage guidelines. It's also a good idea to talk to a healthcare provider before starting any new supplement, especially if you have any underlying health conditions or are taking medications.

How to incorporate beta-glucan into your diet

Adding beta-glucan into diet: There are several ways to incorporate beta-glucan into your diet. Here are some suggestions:

1. Add oats to your breakfast: Oats are one of the best sources of beta-glucan. You can add oats to your breakfast by making oatmeal, overnight oats, or adding oats to your smoothie.
2. Eat barley: Barley is another good source of beta-glucan. You can add cooked barley to salads, soups, stews, or use it as a rice substitute.
3. Choose whole grain products: Whole grains such as whole wheat, brown rice, and quinoa contain beta-glucan. Choose whole grain bread, pasta, and crackers.
4. Snack on nuts and seeds: Nuts and seeds such as almonds, flaxseeds, and chia seeds are also good sources of beta-glucan. You can snack on them or add them to your meals.
5. Consider beta-glucan supplements: Beta-glucan supplements are available in capsules, tablets, and powders. Consult with a healthcare professional before adding supplements to your diet.

Remember that it is important to gradually increase your fiber intake and to drink plenty of water to prevent digestive discomfort. Aim to consume at least 25-30 grams of fiber per day, including sources of beta-glucan.

CHAPTER 3: BETA-GLUCAN AND OBESITY

Beta-glucan, a type of soluble fiber, has been shown to have potential benefits for obesity and weight management.

Beta-glucan and weight management

Research has shown that beta-glucan may be beneficial for weight management.

One way in which beta-glucan may aid in weight management is by promoting feelings of fullness. Studies have found that consuming beta-glucan can increase satiety and reduce hunger, decreasing overall food intake and subsequent weight loss.

Another way in which beta-glucan may contribute to weight management is through its impact on blood sugar levels. Beta-glucan has been shown to slow glucose absorption into the bloodstream, which can help stabilize blood sugar levels and prevent insulin spikes. This can be particularly beneficial for individuals with diabetes or those at risk for developing the condition, as high blood sugar levels can contribute to weight gain and other health problems.

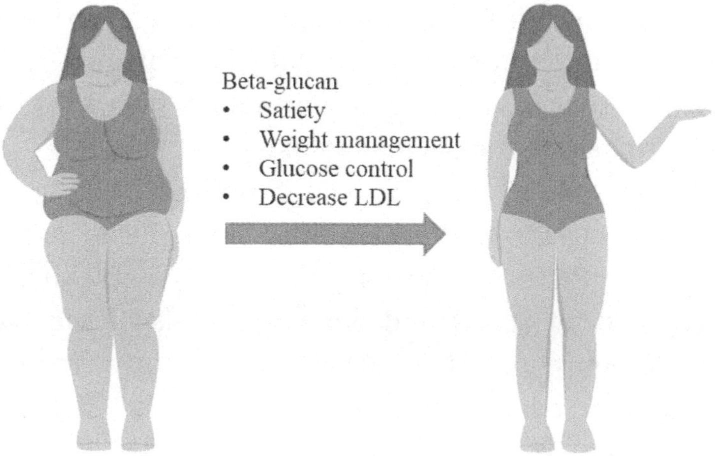

In addition to its effects on satiety and blood sugar levels, beta-glucan may also positively impact gut health. Studies have shown that beta-glucan can help promote the growth of beneficial gut bacteria, which may improve digestion and metabolism.

While beta-glucan alone is unlikely to cause significant weight loss, incorporating foods rich in beta-glucan into a healthy diet may be helpful for those looking to manage their weight or improve their overall health.

Beta-glucan increases satiety

Beta-glucan may regulate appetite and food intake through several mechanisms.

- First, beta-glucan forms a gel-like substance in the stomach when it comes into contact with water. This gel takes up space in the stomach, creating a feeling of fullness and satiety.

- Second, beta-glucan may slow the emptying of the stomach, which can also increase feelings of fullness and reduce hunger. When food stays in the stomach for longer, it can delay the release of hunger hormones such as ghrelin, which can help to reduce food intake.
- Third, beta-glucan may impact hormones that regulate appetite and satiety. For example, beta-glucan has been found to increase levels of the satiety hormone cholecystokinin (CCK) and decrease levels of the hunger hormone ghrelin. This hormonal response can also contribute to reduced food intake.

According to the findings presented by this author's research group, the consumption of oat beta-glucan in humans leads to an increase in the satiety hormone, PYY, in a dose-dependent manner. The colon produces PYY and is responsible for regulating feelings of fullness. The study demonstrated that when beta-glucan was consumed in low (LBG, 2.2g), medium (MBG, 3.8g), and high (HBG, 5.5g) doses, there was a corresponding increase in PYY levels, indicating a dose-response relationship. Therefore, the more beta-glucan is consumed, the more significant the increase in PYY levels.

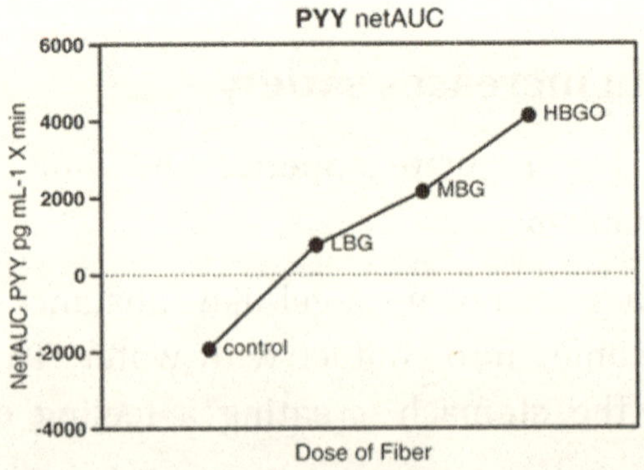

- Beta-glucan may also affect the absorption and metabolism of nutrients in the gut, which can impact appetite and food intake. For example, beta-glucan has been found to slow down the absorption of carbohydrates, which can help to regulate blood sugar levels and reduce hunger.
- Finally, beta-glucan may also affect the microbiome's activity in the gut, which can influence satiety. Some studies have suggested that beta-glucan may promote the growth of beneficial gut bacteria, which can improve gut health and metabolic function. These changes in the gut microbiome may also affect appetite regulation and satiety.

Overall, combining these mechanisms may help regulate appetite and food intake, which can contribute to weight loss and weight management.

Beta-glucan and fat metabolism

Beta-glucan has been found to have several effects on fat metabolism, which can contribute to weight loss and improved metabolic health.

- First, beta-glucan can reduce the absorption of dietary fat in the gut. When beta-glucan forms a gel-like substance in the stomach, it can trap dietary fat and prevent it from being fully absorbed in the small intestine. This means that some of the dietary fat is excreted in the feces, which can lead to reduced calorie intake and weight loss.
- Second, beta-glucan may increase the oxidation of fatty acids, which can lead to increased fat burning and reduced fat storage. This effect is believed to be mediated through an increase in the activity of certain enzymes involved in fatty acid oxidation.

- Third, beta-glucan may improve insulin sensitivity, improving glucose and lipid metabolism. Insulin is a hormone that plays a crucial role in regulating glucose and lipid metabolism, and insulin resistance is a major risk factor for obesity and metabolic disorders. Beta-glucan can improve glucose and lipid metabolism by improving insulin sensitivity and reducing the risk of metabolic diseases.
- Finally, beta-glucan may also have anti-inflammatory effects, which can help to reduce the risk of metabolic disorders such as obesity, type 2 diabetes, and cardiovascular disease. Chronic inflammation is a common feature of these conditions, and reducing inflammation can help to improve metabolic health.

Overall, the effects of beta-glucan on fat metabolism can contribute to weight loss, improved metabolic health, and a reduced risk of metabolic disorders.

CHAPTER 4: BETA-GLUCAN AND METABOLIC SYNDROME

Beta-glucans are soluble dietary fibers in oats, barley, and mushrooms. They have been shown to have health benefits, particularly for metabolic syndrome. Studies suggest that beta-glucans may help improve blood glucose levels, lower cholesterol levels, and improve blood pressure, which are all components of metabolic syndrome. Therefore, beta-glucans may be a beneficial dietary component for individuals with metabolic syndrome.

Beta-glucan and cholesterol

Beta-glucans have been shown to reduce LDL cholesterol levels in various populations, including obese individuals. The cholesterol-lowering effect of beta-glucans is primarily attributed to their soluble fiber content and the way they interact with bile acids in the digestive system. Here's how beta-glucans can help reduce LDL cholesterol in obesity, considering the different types of beta-glucans and their sources:

1. Soluble fiber: Beta-glucans are a type of soluble fiber, meaning they dissolve in water and form a gel-like substance in the digestive system. This property allows them to bind to bile acids, which are compounds synthesized from cholesterol and needed for the digestion and absorption of dietary fats. When beta-glucans bind to bile acids, the resulting complex is excreted from the body. This mechanism reduces the overall amount of cholesterol available for absorption in the intestine and reduces circulating LDL cholesterol levels.

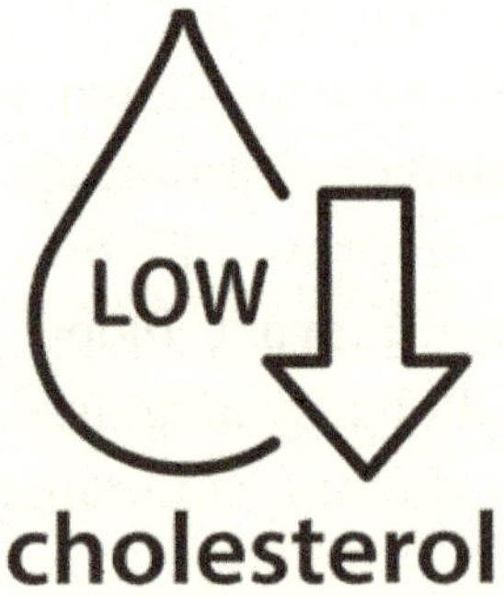

2. Types of beta-glucans: Different types of beta-glucans depend on the source and the structure. The most well-studied sources of beta-glucans with cholesterol-lowering effects are oats and barley. Oat beta-glucans are mainly composed of (1→3),(1→4)-linked β-D-glucopyranosyl units, while barley beta-glucans have a similar structure but with a higher proportion of (1→3)-linkages. These structural differences can influence their solubility, viscosity, and ability to bind bile acids, but

both oat and barley beta-glucans have been shown to be effective in lowering LDL cholesterol.

3. Sources of beta-glucans: As mentioned earlier, oats and barley are the primary sources of beta-glucans with cholesterol-lowering effects. Whole grains, such as oatmeal, rolled oats, and barley flakes, are good dietary beta-glucan sources. Some mushrooms, like shiitake and maitake, also contain beta-glucans. Still, the structure of these beta-glucans is different (primarily (1→3),(1→6)-linked β-D-glucopyranosyl units), and their impact on cholesterol levels is less well established.

In the context of obesity, reducing LDL cholesterol levels is particularly important, as obesity is often associated with dyslipidemia, a condition characterized by elevated LDL cholesterol and other lipid abnormalities. Including beta-glucan sources, such as oats and barley, in a balanced diet can improve lipid profiles in obese individuals. However, addressing other factors, such as overall calorie intake, physical activity, and maintaining a healthy lifestyle, is essential to achieve weight loss and improving cardiovascular health.

Beta-glucan and hypertension

Beta-glucans may benefit hypertension (high blood pressure) in patients with obesity and metabolic syndrome. While the exact mechanisms behind these effects are not yet fully understood, several factors may contribute to the potential blood pressure-lowering effects of beta-glucans in these populations.

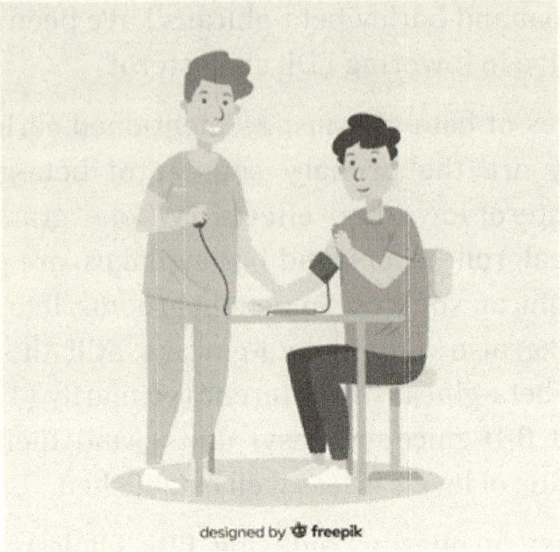

1. Improved insulin sensitivity: Obesity and metabolic syndrome are often characterized by insulin resistance, which can contribute to hypertension. Beta-glucans have been shown to improve insulin sensitivity, which could help regulate blood pressure in these patients.

2. Weight management: Beta-glucans can contribute to a feeling of fullness (satiety) and slow gastric emptying, which may help reduce overall calorie intake and support weight management. Weight loss, even modest amounts, has been shown to positively impact blood pressure in individuals with obesity and metabolic syndrome.

3. Reduced inflammation: Obesity and metabolic syndrome are associated with chronic low-grade inflammation, which can contribute to hypertension. Some research suggests that beta-glucans may have anti-inflammatory properties, which could potentially help reduce blood pressure in these patients.

4. Enhanced nitric oxide production: Nitric oxide is a vasodilator that helps relax and widen blood vessels, thereby reducing blood pressure. Some animal studies have suggested that beta-glucans may increase nitric oxide production, although more research is needed to confirm this effect in humans.

Types of beta-glucans, sources, and doses

There are several types of beta-glucans, but the most commonly studied for their potential health benefits are derived from oats and barley. These sources contain primarily (1,3)(1,4)-beta-D-glucans. Other sources of beta-glucans include certain mushrooms (e.g., shiitake, maitake, and reishi), which contain (1,3)(1,6)-beta-D-glucans.

Doses of beta-glucan may vary depending on the source and the desired health benefits. For example, a daily intake of 3 grams of oat or barley-derived beta-glucan is often recommended for cholesterol-lowering effects, which may indirectly influence blood pressure. However, optimal doses for reducing hypertension are not well established, and more research is needed to determine the most effective dosage.

It is important to note that while beta-glucans may benefit hypertension in individuals with obesity and metabolic syndrome, they should not be considered a substitute for proper medical care and lifestyle modifications. Managing blood pressure typically involves a combination of dietary changes, regular physical activity, weight management, and medication, when needed, under the guidance of a healthcare professional.

Beta-glucan on inflammation

Beta-glucans can help reduce inflammation in obesity and metabolic syndrome through various mechanisms. Different types of beta-glucans and their sources may have distinct properties and effects on inflammation. The primary sources of beta-glucans include cereal grains, such as oats and barley, and certain types of fungi, like mushrooms and yeast.

Here are some potential mechanisms through which beta-glucans may reduce inflammation in obesity and metabolic syndrome:

1. Soluble fiber: Beta-glucans are a type of soluble fiber, which can help lower blood sugar levels, reduce cholesterol, and improve gut health. By regulating blood sugar and lipid levels, beta-glucans can help reduce inflammation associated with obesity and metabolic syndrome.
2. Gut microbiota modulation: Beta-glucans can act as prebiotics, promoting the growth of beneficial gut bacteria, improving gut health, and reducing inflammation. Healthy gut microbiota plays a crucial role in modulating immune responses and reducing systemic inflammation associated with obesity and metabolic syndrome.
3. Direct immune system modulation: Beta-glucans from fungal sources, such as mushrooms and yeast, have been shown to have immunomodulatory properties. They can activate immune cells like macrophages, neutrophils, and natural killer cells, which are essential in controlling inflammation. By modulating the immune response, beta-glucans can help reduce chronic inflammation associated with obesity and metabolic syndrome.

4. Viscosity: The viscosity of beta-glucans in the gut can slow down the digestion and absorption of nutrients, leading to a more gradual increase in blood sugar and insulin levels after a meal. This can help reduce inflammation by preventing rapid blood sugar spikes and the subsequent release of pro-inflammatory molecules.
5. Weight management: As a soluble fiber, beta-glucans can help increase feelings of fullness and satiety, potentially aiding in weight management. Reduced body weight can help alleviate inflammation associated with obesity and metabolic syndrome.

It's important to note that the specific effects of beta-glucans on inflammation can depend on the source, molecular structure, and degree of purity. Further research is needed to fully understand the differences between various types of beta-glucans and their potential benefits in obesity and metabolic syndrome. Nevertheless, incorporating beta-glucan-rich foods into a balanced diet, alongside other anti-inflammatory foods and a healthy lifestyle, can reduce inflammation and improve overall health.

Effects of beta-glucan on type 2 diabetes

Beta-glucan intake can benefit patients with type 2 diabetes for several reasons. Beta-glucans are a type of soluble fiber found in the cell walls of some plants, particularly in oats, barley, and mushrooms. They have been associated with various health benefits, including improving blood sugar control, which is particularly important for people with type 2 diabetes. Here are some reasons why beta-glucan intake can be helpful for these patients:

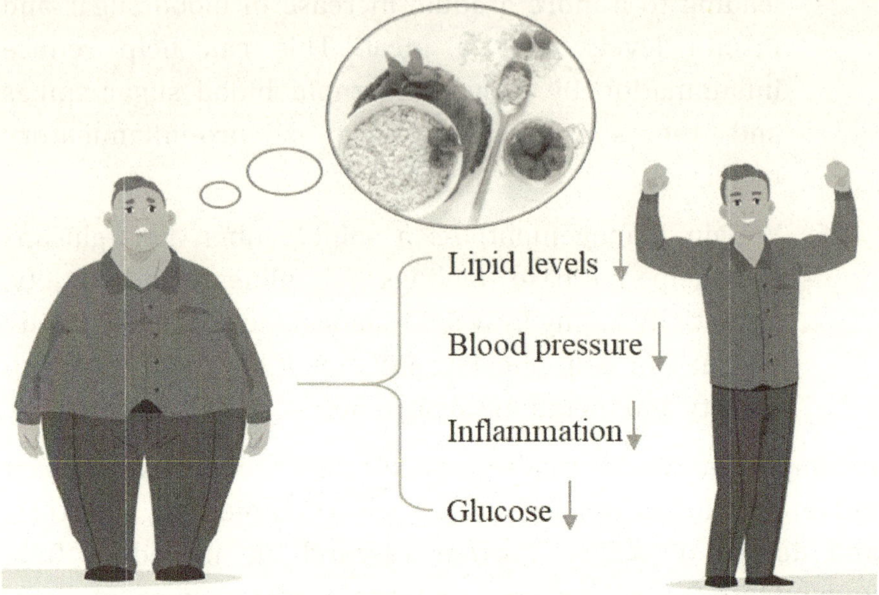

1. Improved glycemic control: Beta-glucans slow down glucose absorption in the digestive tract, which helps to maintain more stable blood sugar levels. This reduces postprandial (after-meal) glucose and insulin spikes, improving overall glycemic control.
2. Increased insulin sensitivity: Some studies have shown that regular consumption of beta-glucans can improve insulin sensitivity, which means that the body can better use insulin to regulate blood sugar levels. Improved insulin sensitivity can help to prevent or manage type 2 diabetes.
3. Reduced appetite and weight management: Beta-glucans can increase the feeling of fullness (satiety) and slow down gastric emptying, which may help to reduce

overall calorie intake and support weight management. Maintaining a healthy weight is important for people with type 2 diabetes, as excess body weight is a risk factor for developing and progressing the disease.

4. Lower cholesterol levels: Beta-glucans have been shown to reduce LDL cholesterol levels ("bad" cholesterol) and improve overall lipid profiles. High LDL cholesterol levels are a risk factor for cardiovascular disease, which is more common in people with type 2 diabetes.
5. Anti-inflammatory effects: Some research suggests that beta-glucans may have anti-inflammatory properties, which could be beneficial for individuals with type 2 diabetes, as chronic inflammation is associated with the development and progression of the disease.

It's important to note that while beta-glucans can have positive effects on blood sugar control and other aspects of health, they should not be considered a substitute for proper medical care and management of type 2 diabetes. Individuals with diabetes should work closely with their healthcare provider to develop a comprehensive treatment plan that includes a balanced diet, regular physical activity, and appropriate medication, if necessary.

CHAPTER 5: BETA-GLUCAN AND HEART HEALTH

Dietary fiber and heart health

Fiber plays an important role in heart health. Here are some ways in which fiber can help:

1. Lowers cholesterol levels: Soluble fiber, such as beta-glucan, can help lower cholesterol levels by reducing cholesterol absorption in the intestines. This can help reduce the risk of heart disease.

2. Reduces blood pressure: Eating a diet high in fiber can help lower blood pressure. This is because fiber helps regulate blood sugar levels, which in turn can lower blood pressure.

3. Reduces inflammation: Inflammation is a risk factor for heart disease. Eating a diet high in fiber can help reduce inflammation in the body.

4. Improves gut health: A healthy gut microbiome is important for overall health, including heart health. Fiber helps promote the growth of beneficial gut bacteria, which can positively impact heart health.

5. Helps with weight management: A diet high in fiber can help with weight management. This is because fiber helps you feel full, so you are less likely to overeat.

Healty Heart

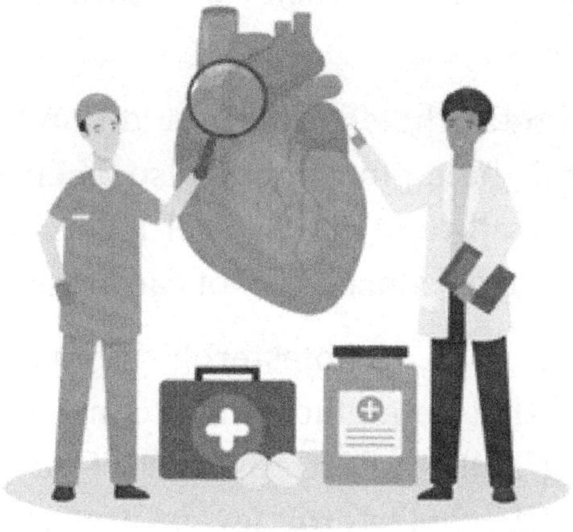

Therefore, consuming a diet high in fiber can have numerous benefits for heart health. It is recommended to consume at least 25-30 grams of fiber per day, including various fiber sources such as whole grains, fruits, vegetables, legumes, nuts, and seeds.

Beta-glucan and heart health

Beta-glucan has been shown to have several beneficial effects on heart health, primarily through its impact on cholesterol levels and its potential anti-inflammatory properties. Here are some ways in which beta-glucan intake can promote heart health:

1. Lowering LDL cholesterol: Beta-glucan can bind to bile acids in the digestive tract, which are then excreted from the body. As bile acids are synthesized from cholesterol, the liver must use more cholesterol to produce new bile acids, ultimately reducing LDL cholesterol levels ("bad" cholesterol). High LDL cholesterol levels are a major risk factor for atherosclerosis and cardiovascular disease development.

2. Reducing total cholesterol: In addition to lowering LDL cholesterol, beta-glucan has also been shown to help reduce overall total cholesterol levels. This can further contribute to a reduced risk of cardiovascular disease.

3. Improving HDL cholesterol: Some studies have suggested that beta-glucan intake may positively impact increasing HDL cholesterol levels ("good" cholesterol). Higher HDL cholesterol levels are associated with a lower risk of cardiovascular disease, as HDL helps remove excess cholesterol from the bloodstream and transport it back to the liver for elimination.

4. Anti-inflammatory effects: Chronic inflammation is a contributing factor in the development of atherosclerosis and cardiovascular disease. Some research has indicated that beta-glucans may have anti-inflammatory properties, which could potentially help reduce the risk of heart-related issues.

5. Blood pressure reduction: Although the evidence is not as strong as for cholesterol-lowering effects, some studies have suggested that beta-glucan may have a modest impact on lowering blood pressure. High blood pressure is another risk factor for cardiovascular disease.

To reap the heart health benefits of beta-glucan, it is important to consume a diet that is rich in whole grains, such as oats and barley, and include other sources of beta-glucan, such as certain mushrooms. However, it is essential to remember that maintaining good heart health involves more than just beta-glucan intake. A balanced diet, regular physical activity, stress management, and avoiding smoking are all crucial components of a heart-healthy lifestyle.

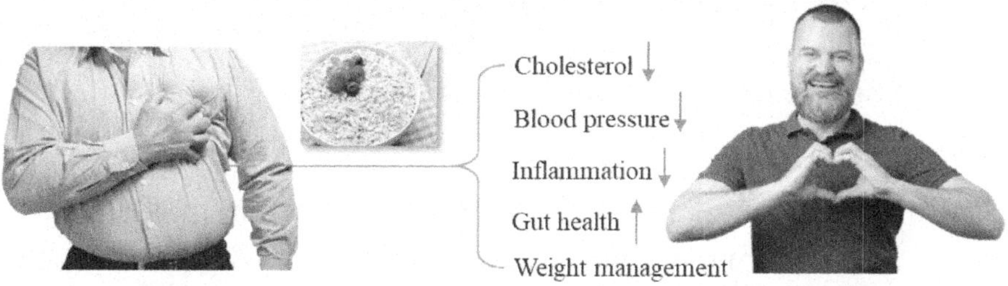

Cardiovascular disease

Improve heart health

Compare beta-glucan with other dietary fibers

Beta-glucans and other dietary fibers can offer heart health benefits through various mechanisms. Comparing beta-glucan effects with other dietary fibers can help clarify their unique and shared benefits. Here is an overview of the heart health benefits of beta-glucans and some other common dietary fibers:

1. Beta-glucans:

- Source: Primarily found in oats, barley, and certain mushrooms.
- Mechanism: Beta-glucans are soluble fibers that form a gel-like substance in the digestive tract, binding to bile acids and promoting their excretion. This leads to a

reduction in LDL cholesterol levels, as the liver needs to use more cholesterol to produce new bile acids. Beta-glucans have also been associated with anti-inflammatory effects and may have a modest impact on blood pressure regulation.

- Heart health benefits: Reduced LDL cholesterol levels, improved overall lipid profile, potential anti-inflammatory effects, and possible blood pressure reduction.

2. Psyllium:

- Source: Derived from the seeds of the Plantago ovate plant.
- Mechanism: Psyllium is a soluble fiber that, like beta-glucans, forms a gel-like substance in the digestive tract. This gel binds to bile acids and cholesterol, helping to lower cholesterol levels. Psyllium may also slow down glucose absorption, thereby improving blood sugar control.
- Heart health benefits: Reduced LDL cholesterol levels, improved overall lipid profile, and better blood sugar control.

3. Pectin:

- Source: Found in the cell walls of many fruits, including apples, pears, and citrus fruits.
- Mechanism: Pectin is another soluble fiber that binds to bile acids and cholesterol in the digestive tract. It has also been suggested to help reduce inflammation and improve blood sugar control.

- Heart health benefits: Reduced LDL cholesterol levels, potential anti-inflammatory effects, and better blood sugar control.

4. Inulin:

- Source: Found in various plant foods, including chicory root, Jerusalem artichoke, onions, and garlic.
- Mechanism: Inulin is a prebiotic soluble fiber that supports the growth of beneficial gut bacteria. This can produce short-chain fatty acids, which may help regulate cholesterol synthesis in the liver and reduce inflammation.
- Heart health benefits: Potential reduction in cholesterol levels and anti-inflammatory effects.

5. Cellulose:

- Source: Found in the cell walls of many plant foods, including whole grains, fruits, and vegetables.
- Mechanism: Cellulose is an insoluble fiber that helps promote bowel regularity and adds bulk to the diet. While it does not directly lower cholesterol levels, consuming a diet rich in insoluble fiber can support overall heart health by promoting a healthy weight and improving blood sugar control.
- Heart health benefits include improved bowel regularity, weight management, and control of blood sugar.

While each of these dietary fibers has unique mechanisms of action, they all contribute to heart health in various ways. Incorporating a mix of soluble and insoluble fibers from diverse sources is crucial for maintaining good cardiovascular health, as they offer complementary benefits. A balanced diet, rich in whole grains, fruits, vegetables, and legumes, can help provide an adequate intake of these essential fibers.

Doses and forms of beta-glucan

The impact of different doses and forms of beta-glucans on heart health outcomes can vary, with factors such as source, individual response, and overall diet playing a role. Here is an overview of the effects of whole foods, supplements, and functional foods containing beta-glucans:

1. Whole foods:

- Sources: Oats, barley, and certain mushrooms are natural sources of beta-glucans.
- Impact: Consuming whole foods containing beta-glucans as part of a balanced diet can provide additional nutrients, such as vitamins, minerals, and other dietary fibers. These nutrients can work synergistically to improve heart health. Whole food sources are usually well-tolerated and have lower adverse effects and risks than supplements.
- Doses: The recommended daily intake of beta-glucans for cholesterol-lowering effects is about 3 grams. This can be achieved by consuming around 1.5 cups of cooked oatmeal or a similar serving of barley.

2. Supplements:

- Sources: Beta-glucan supplements are usually derived from oats, barley, or certain mushrooms.
- Impact: Supplements can provide a concentrated source of beta-glucans and may be useful for individuals who have difficulty incorporating whole food sources into

their diets. However, they may not provide the additional nutrients and benefits associated with whole foods. Moreover, supplements can potentially interact with medications or cause adverse effects, so it is essential to consult a healthcare professional before using them.

- Doses: The optimal dosage for beta-glucan supplements depends on the specific product and the desired health outcome. Following the manufacturer's guidelines and consulting a healthcare professional for personalized advice is essential.

3. Functional foods:

- Sources: Functional foods containing beta-glucans include fortified cereals, bread, yogurt, and beverages.
- Impact: These products can help increase beta-glucan intake for individuals who may not consume sufficient amounts through whole food sources. However, it is important to consider the overall nutritional quality of functional foods, as some may also contain added sugars, sodium, or unhealthy fats that could counteract the heart health benefits of beta-glucans.
- Doses: The amount of beta-glucans in functional foods can vary widely, so it is essential to read product labels and determine the contribution of these foods to the recommended daily intake.

In summary, incorporating beta-glucans into the diet through various forms can impact heart health outcomes differently. Whole foods are generally the best option, as they provide additional nutrients and benefits. However, supplements and functional foods can also play a role in certain circumstances. It is important to consult a healthcare professional for personalized advice and consider the overall nutritional quality of the diet when including beta-glucans from different sources.

Synergistic effects

The synergistic effects of beta-glucans and other heart-healthy nutrients, such as omega-3 fatty acids and antioxidants, can contribute to improved cardiovascular health. Each nutrient offers unique benefits, and when combined, they may work together to promote overall heart health more effectively than when consumed individually. Here are some ways these nutrients can work together:

1. Beta-glucans and omega-3 fatty acids:

- Beta-glucans help lower LDL cholesterol levels and may modestly reduce blood pressure.
- Omega-3 fatty acids, particularly EPA and DHA found in fatty fish, can reduce inflammation, lower triglyceride levels, and help prevent blood clot formation.
- Synergistic effects: Consuming both beta-glucans and omega-3 fatty acids can comprehensively manage cholesterol levels, reduce inflammation, and promote overall cardiovascular health.

2. Beta-glucans and plant-based antioxidants:

- Plant-based antioxidants, such as flavonoids found in berries, cocoa, and green tea, can help protect LDL cholesterol from oxidation, reduce inflammation, and improve endothelial function (blood vessel health).
- Synergistic effects: Combining beta-glucans with antioxidant-rich foods can help lower LDL cholesterol levels while providing additional protection against

oxidative damage and inflammation associated with cardiovascular disease development.

3. Beta-glucans and other heart-healthy nutrients:

- Nutrients such as magnesium, potassium, and fiber found in whole grains, fruits, vegetables, and legumes can help regulate blood pressure, support heart muscle function, and maintain healthy cholesterol levels.
- Synergistic effects: Including beta-glucans in a diet rich in a variety of heart-healthy nutrients can further support cardiovascular health by targeting multiple risk factors, such as high cholesterol, high blood pressure, and inflammation.

To maximize the synergistic effects of beta-glucans and other heart-healthy nutrients, consider the following dietary approaches:

- Consume a diet rich in whole grains, fruits, vegetables, legumes, nuts, and seeds to ensure a variety of fiber types, antioxidants, and essential minerals.
- Include sources of omega-3 fatty acids, such as fatty fish (salmon, mackerel, sardines), walnuts, chia seeds, and flaxseeds.
- Opt for antioxidant-rich foods like berries, dark chocolate, and green tea to provide additional protection against oxidative stress and inflammation.

By incorporating a diverse range of heart-healthy nutrients in the diet, including beta-glucans, individuals can support their cardiovascular health more effectively than relying on a single nutrient or dietary component. In addition, a balanced, nutrient-rich diet, regular physical activity, and other healthy lifestyle habits are vital to maintaining good heart health.

Beta-glucan rich foods

Incorporating beta-glucan-rich foods into a heart-healthy diet can be simple and enjoyable. Here are some dietary recommendations and practical tips to help you include more beta-glucans in your daily meals:

1. Choose whole grains:

- Opt for oats and barley as your primary whole grain sources since they are rich in beta-glucans. This can include steel-cut oats, old-fashioned oats, quick oats, oat bran, barley flakes, and pearled barley.

2. Breakfast ideas:

- Start your day with a bowl of oatmeal, adding berries, nuts, and seeds for extra flavor and nutrition.
- Make overnight oats by combining rolled oats with milk or yogurt and refrigerate overnight. Add your favorite fruit, nuts, and a drizzle of honey or maple syrup in the morning.
- Prepare muesli by mixing oats, dried fruits, nuts, and seeds. Serve with milk, yogurt, or as a topping for fresh fruit.

3. Soups and stews:

- Add barley or oats to soups and stews to increase their beta-glucan content. Barley works well in vegetable, chicken, and beef-based soups, while oats can be used as a thickener in creamy soups.

4. Baking and cooking:

- Use oat flour or oat bran as a partial replacement for all-purpose flour in bread, muffins, pancakes, or cookies recipes.
- Make a savory barley risotto using pearled barley instead of rice for a beta-glucan-rich twist on the classic dish.

5. Snacks and sides:

- Incorporate beta-glucan-rich foods into your snacks by choosing oat-based granola bars or whole-grain crackers made with oats or barley.
- Prepare a barley salad with mixed vegetables, legumes, and your favorite salad dressing for a healthy side dish.

6. Explore mushroom varieties:

- Add mushrooms like shiitake, maitake, and reishi, which contain beta-glucans, to stir-fries, pasta dishes, soups, or salads.

7. Read food labels:

- When purchasing packaged foods like cereal, bread, or crackers, read the labels and look for products made with whole oats or barley. Be cautious about added sugars, sodium, and unhealthy fats.

8. Gradual introduction:

- If you're not accustomed to eating oats, barley, or mushrooms, start by introducing them gradually to your diet to give your digestive system time to adapt.

Remember that a heart-healthy diet is about more than just beta-glucans. Be sure to include a variety of fruits, vegetables, lean proteins, healthy fats, and other whole grains in your daily meals to ensure a balanced and diverse nutrient intake.

Combine this with regular physical activity, stress management, and adequate sleep to promote optimal heart health.

Meals rich in beta-glucan to support heart health

Incorporating meals like these into your diet can help increase your intake of beta-glucans and other heart-healthy nutrients, thereby supporting cardiovascular health. Here are two meal examples rich in beta-glucans to support heart health:

Breakfast

Imagine a warm, comforting bowl of oatmeal with a slightly creamy texture. The surface of the oatmeal is topped with a colorful mix of fresh berries, including blueberries, strawberries, and raspberries. Chopped nuts, such as walnuts or almonds, are sprinkled over the berries, adding a crunchy texture. A small pile of chia seeds sits on top, and a drizzle of honey or maple syrup glistens as it drapes over the entire dish.

Receips:

Breakfast - Oatmeal with Berries, Nuts, and Chia Seeds

- 1.5 cups cooked old-fashioned or steel-cut oats (provides around 3 grams of beta-glucans)
- 1/2 cup mixed berries (e.g., blueberries, strawberries, raspberries)
- 1/4 cup chopped nuts (e.g., walnuts or almonds)
- 1 tablespoon chia seeds
- A drizzle of honey or maple syrup (optional)

Instructions: Cook the oats according to package instructions or prepare overnight oats as mentioned earlier. If desired, top with mixed berries, chopped nuts, chia seeds, and a drizzle of honey or maple syrup. This meal provides a good amount of beta-glucans from oats, healthy fats, fiber, and antioxidants from berries, nuts, and chia seeds.

Dinner

Picture a colorful stir-fry with an array of bright vegetables like bell peppers, broccoli, carrots, and snap peas, cooked to tender-crisp perfection. The vegetables are mixed with tender, cooked pearled barley with a slightly chewy texture and a mild, nutty flavor. The dish is seasoned with fragrant garlic and ginger, and a touch of low-sodium soy sauce lends a savory, umami taste. Beside the stir-fry on the plate is a beautifully grilled salmon fillet with a golden, slightly crispy exterior and a tender, flaky interior.

Receips:

Dinner Barley and Vegetable Stir-Fry with Grilled Salmon

- 1 cup cooked pearled barley (provides around 2-3 grams of beta-glucans)
- 2 cups mixed vegetables (e.g., bell peppers, broccoli, carrots, snap peas)
- 1 tablespoon olive oil
- 1/4 cup low-sodium soy sauce or tamari
- 1 tablespoon minced garlic
- 1 tablespoon minced ginger

- 4 oz grilled salmon (provides heart-healthy omega-3 fatty acids)

Instructions: Cook pearled barley according to package instructions. Heat the olive oil and add garlic and ginger in a large skillet or wok. Sauté for 1-2 minutes until fragrant. Add the mixed vegetables and cook until tender-crisp. Stir in the cooked barley and low-sodium soy sauce, cooking for another 2-3 minutes until heated.

Serve the barley and vegetable stir-fry alongside a 4 oz portion of grilled salmon. This meal offers beta-glucans from the barley, various vegetable nutrients, and omega-3 fatty acids from the salmon.

CHAPTER 6: BETA-GLUCAN AND IMMUNE HEALTH

Introduction

Immunity is the body's natural defense mechanism that helps protect us from infections, diseases, and harmful substances. It plays a crucial role in maintaining health and overall well-being. Our immune system consists of a complex network of cells, tissues, and organs that work together to recognize and neutralize foreign substances, such as bacteria, viruses, fungi, parasites, and abnormal or damaged cells, like cancerous cells.

The immune system has two primary components: innate immunity and adaptive immunity. First, innate immunity is our first line of defense and involves non-specific, rapid responses to a wide range of pathogens. This includes physical barriers like skin and mucous membranes and immune cells such as macrophages, neutrophils, and natural killer (NK) cells. Second, adaptive immunity, on the other hand, is a more specialized and targeted response involving immune cells like B and T lymphocytes. Adaptive immunity develops over time as our immune system encounters and remembers specific pathogens, providing long-lasting protection against future infections.

A healthy immune system is essential for survival, allowing us to fight off infections and recover from illnesses more effectively. Conversely, a weakened or compromised immune system can increase susceptibility to infections and a higher risk of developing chronic diseases. Therefore, maintaining a strong and well-functioning immune system is vital for overall health and well-being. This can be achieved through a balanced diet, regular exercise, adequate sleep, stress management, and other healthy lifestyle habits.

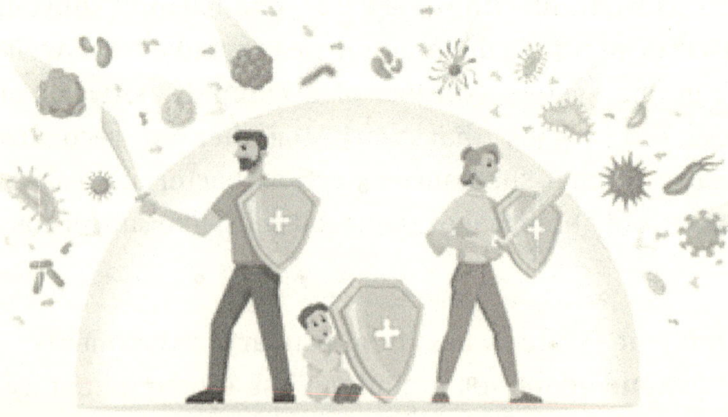

Immune-modulating effects

Beta-glucans are a type of naturally occurring polysaccharide with immune-modulating properties. These complex carbohydrates are glucose molecules linked together by βglycosidic bonds, giving them their unique structure and function. Beta-glucans can be found in various sources such as the cell walls of yeast, fungi (including mushrooms), and cereals like oats and barley.

The immune-modulating effects of beta-glucans have gained considerable interest in recent years due to their potential benefits in supporting and enhancing the immune system. Research has shown that beta-glucans can interact with immune cells, such as macrophages, neutrophils, and dendritic cells, influencing their activity and function. These interactions can lead to the activation of immune cell receptors, stimulation of cytokine production, and enhancement of both innate and adaptive immune responses.

As a result, beta-glucans have been explored for their potential applications in various health contexts, such as improving immunity against infections, supporting the immune response in cancer therapy, and acting as adjuvants in vaccines. Although research is still ongoing, the immune-modulating properties of beta-glucans hold promise for their potential use as dietary supplements or functional food ingredients to support overall immune health.

Beta-glucans interact with immune cells

Beta-glucans interact with immune cells by binding to specific cell surface receptors, which initiates a cascade of signaling events that modulate the immune response. The primary immune cells that interact with beta-glucans include macrophages, neutrophils, and dendritic cells, all of which play essential roles in the innate immune system.

1. Macrophages: These cells are responsible for phagocytosis or engulfing and digesting foreign particles, pathogens, and cellular debris. Beta-glucans can bind to receptors like dectin-1 and complement receptor 3 (CR3) on the surface of macrophages. This binding triggers a signaling pathway that activates the macrophage and enhances its ability to destroy pathogens, produce cytokines, and stimulate other immune cells.
2. Neutrophils: These are the most abundant type of white blood cells and are the first responders to infection. Beta-glucans can also bind to CR3 receptors on neutrophils, increasing their ability to migrate to the site of infection, produce reactive oxygen species (ROS), and eliminate pathogens through phagocytosis.
3. Dendritic cells act as messengers between the innate and adaptive immune systems, helping generate a targeted immune response. When dendritic cells encounter beta-glucans, they can internalize and process them, activating cell surface receptors like dectin-1. This activation induces the maturation of dendritic cells, increasing their expression of major histocompatibility complex (MHC) molecules and costimulatory molecules, which are essential for presenting antigens to T cells and initiating an adaptive immune response.

The interaction of beta-glucans with these immune cells leads to a series of signaling events that enhance immune cell function, promote the production of cytokines and chemokines, and stimulate both innate and adaptive immune responses. This immune modulation may contribute to beta-glucans' potential health benefits, such as improving infection resistance and supporting immune function in various clinical contexts.

Beta-glucans enhance immune function

Beta-glucans have been studied for their potential applications in enhancing immune function in various contexts, such as infection, vaccination, and cancer therapy. Here are some of the possible applications:

1. Infection: Beta-glucans have been shown to enhance immune function and improve resistance to bacterial, viral, and fungal infections. Their ability to modulate the immune response, stimulate cytokine production, and activate immune cells like macrophages, neutrophils, and dendritic cells can help the body mount a more effective defense against pathogens. Beta-glucans may also have a role in reducing the severity of infections and improving recovery times.
2. Vaccination: Beta-glucans have been studied as potential adjuvants in vaccines, which are substances that enhance the body's immune response to a vaccine antigen. By stimulating the immune system and promoting the activation of antigen-presenting cells like dendritic cells, beta-glucans may help improve the efficacy of vaccines and induce stronger, longer-lasting immune responses. This has been explored in the context of both bacterial and viral vaccines.
3. Cancer therapy: Beta-glucans have shown potential as immunomodulatory agents in cancer treatment. They can enhance the body's immune response against cancer cells by activating immune cells like macrophages, natural killer (NK) cells, and cytotoxic T cells, which are involved in recognizing and destroying tumor cells. In

addition, beta-glucans have also been found to stimulate the production of cytokines that support anti-tumor immunity. In some cases, they have been studied as adjuncts to conventional cancer treatments, such as chemotherapy and radiation therapy, to improve treatment outcomes and reduce side effects.

While research on beta-glucans and their potential applications in immune function enhancement is still ongoing, these studies demonstrate the promising role that beta-glucans may play in supporting the immune system in various health contexts. Further research is needed to establish optimal dosages, administration methods, and specific beta-glucan sources for each application.

Obesity and metabolic syndrome Immunity

Obesity and metabolic syndrome are closely related conditions that can negatively impact immunity and increase the risk of various health problems. Obesity is characterized by excessive body fat accumulation, while metabolic syndrome refers to a cluster of conditions, including abdominal obesity, high blood pressure, elevated blood sugar, high triglycerides, and low high-density lipoprotein (HDL) cholesterol levels. Both obesity and metabolic syndrome are associated with chronic low-grade inflammation, which can impair immune function.

Here are some ways obesity and metabolic syndrome can affect immunity:

1. Chronic inflammation: Excess adipose tissue, particularly visceral fat, can produce pro-inflammatory cytokines and adipokines, contributing to a chronic low-grade inflammatory state. This persistent inflammation

can disrupt the normal functioning of the immune system and increase the risk of developing various health problems, such as cardiovascular disease and type 2 diabetes.

2. Impaired immune cell function: Obesity and metabolic syndrome can negatively affect the function of various immune cells, including macrophages, neutrophils, and lymphocytes. This can lead to an impaired immune response and a reduced ability to fight off infections.
3. Increased susceptibility to infections: Individuals with obesity or metabolic syndrome may be more susceptible to bacterial, viral, and fungal infections due to the altered immune response. They may also experience more severe symptoms and longer recovery times.
4. Reduced vaccine effectiveness: Some studies have suggested that obesity might be associated with a reduced immune response to certain vaccinations, potentially resulting in lower vaccine effectiveness in individuals with obesity.
5. Impaired wound healing: Obesity and metabolic syndrome can result in impaired wound healing due to a combination of factors, including reduced immune cell function, decreased blood flow, and increased inflammation.

Managing obesity and metabolic syndrome can help improve immune function and overall health. This can be achieved through lifestyle modifications, such as adopting a balanced diet, engaging in regular physical activity, maintaining a healthy weight, getting adequate sleep, and managing stress. In some cases, medical intervention may be necessary to address underlying conditions contributing to obesity or metabolic syndrome.

Effects on obesity Immunity

Beta-glucans have been studied for their potential effects on obesity and metabolic syndrome and their impact on immunity in the context of these conditions. Here are some ways in which beta-glucans may influence obesity, metabolic syndrome, and immunity:

1. Reducing inflammation: Beta-glucans have been shown to possess anti-inflammatory properties, which may help counteract the chronic low-grade inflammation associated with obesity and metabolic syndrome. Beta-glucans may improve immune function and overall health in individuals with these conditions by reducing inflammation.

2. Modulating gut microbiota: Research suggests that beta-glucans can promote the growth of beneficial gut bacteria, which play a crucial role in maintaining gut health and modulating the immune system. A healthy gut microbiota has been linked to reduced inflammation and improved immune function, which could benefit individuals with obesity and metabolic syndrome.

3. Improving glycemic control: Beta-glucans, particularly those derived from oats and barley, have been shown to improve glycemic control by slowing down the absorption of carbohydrates and reducing postprandial blood glucose levels. Better glycemic control can help manage metabolic syndrome and reduce the risk of type 2 diabetes, which may positively affect immune function.

4. Supporting weight management: Some research suggests that beta-glucans may help with weight management by promoting satiety and reducing calorie intake. This could contribute to weight loss or maintaining a healthy weight, which is crucial for managing obesity and metabolic syndrome and improving immune function.

5. Enhancing immune function: As discussed earlier, beta-glucans can interact with immune cells, such as macrophages, neutrophils, and dendritic cells, and modulate immune responses. In the context of obesity and metabolic syndrome, this immune modulation may help improve the overall immune function and resistance to infections.

While the research on beta-glucans and their impact on obesity, metabolic syndrome, and immunity is promising, further studies are needed to establish the optimal sources, doses, and forms of beta-glucans for these applications. Incorporating beta-glucan-rich foods, such as oats and barley, into a balanced diet and other healthy lifestyle habits may contribute to improved immune function and overall health in individuals with obesity and metabolic syndrome.

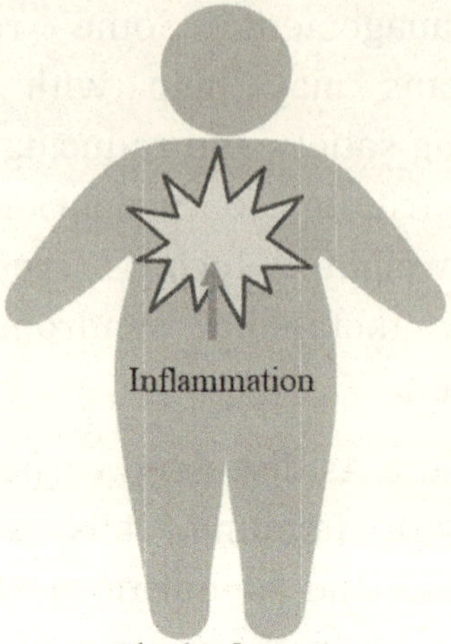

Obesity features a
low-grade inflammation

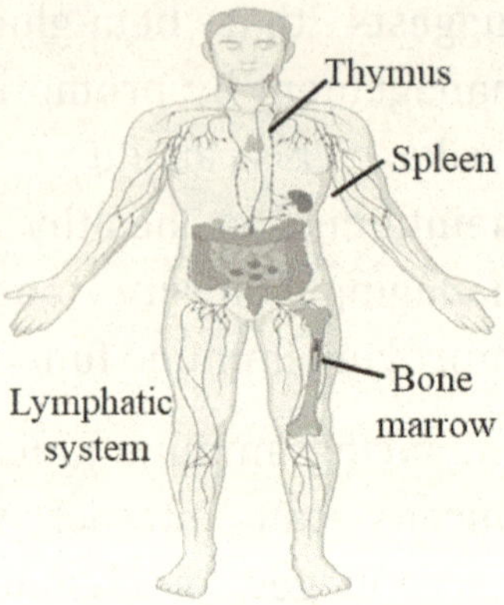

Body immune system

Research has shown that a diet rich in fiber can help to reduce the risk of certain diseases, such as colorectal cancer and type 2 diabetes, which are associated with impaired immune function. Therefore, consuming adequate amounts of fiber as part of a healthy diet is important to support immune health.

Meal to boost immunity

Here are two meal examples rich in beta-glucans that can help boost immunity for individuals with obesity and metabolic syndrome:

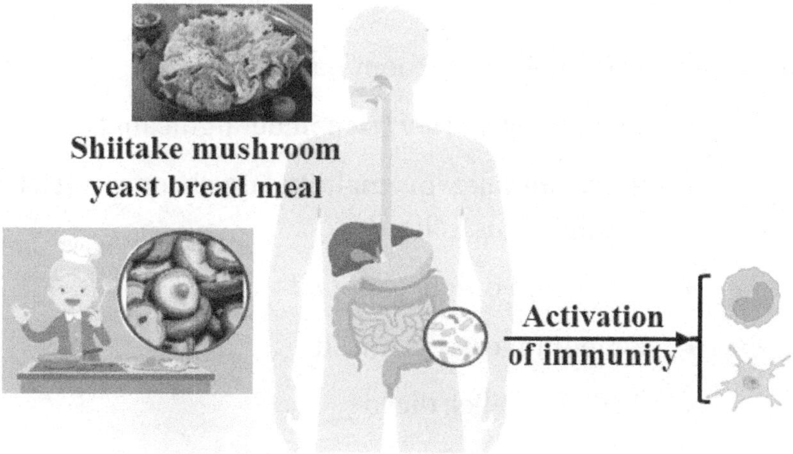

Meal 1:

- Breakfast: Overnight Oats with Berries and Nuts
    - 1/2 cup rolled oats (rich in beta-glucans)
    - 1 cup unsweetened almond milk or low-fat milk
    - 1/2 cup mixed berries (e.g., blueberries, raspberries, and strawberries)
    - 1 tbsp chia seeds
    - 1 tbsp chopped nuts (e.g., almonds, walnuts, or pecans)
    - Optional: a drizzle of honey or a pinch of cinnamon for added flavor

Combine rolled oats, milk, and chia seeds in a mason jar or airtight container, and refrigerate overnight. In the morning, top with mixed berries, chopped nuts, and any additional desired toppings.

Meal 2:

- Lunch or Dinner: Mushroom Barley Soup
    - 1 cup pearl barley (rich in beta-glucans)
    - 8 oz shiitake or maitake mushrooms (rich in beta-glucans), sliced
    - 1 medium onion, chopped
    - 2 medium carrots, diced
    - 2 celery stalks, diced
    - 4 cups low-sodium vegetable broth
    - 2 cups water
    - 2 cloves garlic, minced
    - 1 tbsp olive oil
    - Salt and pepper, to taste
    - Optional: fresh herbs (e.g., parsley, thyme) for garnish

In a large pot, heat olive oil over medium heat. Add onions, carrots, and celery, and cook until softened. Add garlic and cook for an additional minute. Stir in mushrooms, barley, vegetable broth, and water. Bring to a boil, then reduce heat and let simmer for 45-60 minutes or until the barley is tender. Season with salt and pepper to taste. Serve hot, garnished with fresh herbs if desired.

These meal examples provide a good source of beta-glucans from oats, barley, and mushrooms, along with other immune-boosting nutrients such as antioxidants, vitamins, and minerals. Incorporating these meals into a balanced diet, along with regular exercise, adequate sleep, and stress management, can help support immune function and overall health for individuals with obesity and metabolic syndrome.

CHAPTER 7: BETA-GLUCAN AND GUT HEALTH

One way in which beta-glucans may support gut health is by acting as a prebiotic, meaning that they provide food for beneficial gut bacteria. This can help promote the growth of these bacteria, which can help support a healthy gut microbiome. A healthy gut microbiome is vital for digestion, nutrient absorption, and immune system function.

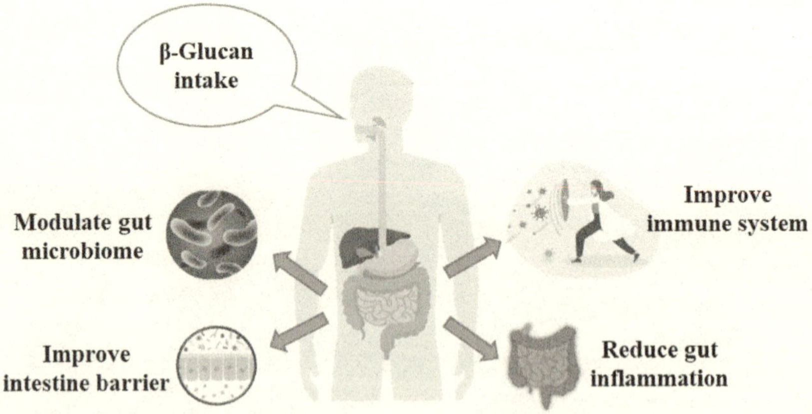

Beta-glucans may also help to improve gut barrier function. The gut barrier comprises a layer of cells that helps prevent harmful substances from entering the body. If the gut barrier becomes damaged, this can lead to inflammation and other health problems. Research has suggested that beta-glucans may help to strengthen the gut barrier, which can help to prevent these issues.

In addition, beta-glucans may help to reduce inflammation in the gut. Chronic inflammation in the gut can contribute to a range of health problems, including inflammatory bowel disease (IBD). Research has suggested that beta-glucans may help reduce gut inflammation by modulating the immune system.

Beta-glucan fermentation by gut bacteria

Beta-glucans are complex polysaccharides that are found in the cell walls of various organisms, including bacteria, fungi, and plants. Humans do not digest these polysaccharides; therefore, they pass through the small intestine undigested and are fermented by the gut microbiota in the large intestine.

The fermentation of beta-glucans by gut bacteria involves a complex series of biochemical reactions that are carried out by different microbial species. The primary mechanism of beta-glucan fermentation involves the breakdown of the polysaccharides into smaller sugar molecules by the action of enzymes produced by the gut bacteria. These enzymes include beta-glucosidases, which cleave the beta-glucan molecule at specific sites, releasing glucose molecules.

Once the beta-glucans are broken down into smaller sugar molecules, they are metabolized by different gut bacterial species. Some of the major bacterial groups involved in beta-glucan fermentation include Bacteroides, Prevotella, and Firmicutes. These bacteria use the sugar molecules released from beta-glucans as a source of energy, producing short-chain fatty acids (SCFAs) such as butyrate, acetate, and propionate. These SCFAs play important roles in maintaining gut health by promoting beneficial bacteria growth and suppressing harmful bacteria growth.

In addition to producing SCFAs, gut bacteria also produce other metabolites during beta-glucan fermentation, including gases such as hydrogen, carbon dioxide, and methane, as well as other organic acids such as lactate and succinate.

Overall, the fermentation of beta-glucans by gut bacteria is an important process that contributes to maintaining gut health and regulating metabolic and immune functions.

Gut bacteria for beta-glucan fermentation

Beta-glucans are complex carbohydrates that are found in various sources such as yeast, fungi, and certain grains like oats and barley. Several gut bacteria are involved in the fermentation of beta-glucans, which results in the production of short-chain fatty acids (SCFAs) such as acetate, propionate, and butyrate.

Some of the common types of gut bacteria that are involved in beta-glucan fermentation include:

1. Bifidobacterium: This group of bacteria is known for its ability to ferment various carbohydrates, including beta-glucans. Bifidobacterium produces acetate, lactate, and other organic acids during fermentation.

2. Lactobacillus: Another group of bacteria that is commonly found in the gut and is involved in beta-glucan fermentation is Lactobacillus. This group of bacteria is also known for its ability to produce lactic acid during fermentation.
3. Bacteroides: Bacteroides are a group of bacteria that are known to ferment various carbohydrates, including beta-glucans. These bacteria produce acetate, propionate, and butyrate as the end products of fermentation.
4. Prevotella: Prevotella is another group of bacteria that are known to be involved in the fermentation of beta-glucans. Like Bacteroides, Prevotella produces acetate, propionate, and butyrate as the end products of fermentation.

In summary, the fermentation of beta-glucans by gut bacteria produces SCFAs such as acetate, propionate, and butyrate. The types of bacteria involved in this process include Bifidobacterium, Lactobacillus, Bacteroides, and Prevotella.

Factors influence the fermentation

The fermentation of beta-glucans in the gut is influenced by several factors, including diet, gut microbiota composition, and gut dysbiosis.

1. Diet: The type and amount of beta-glucans consumed in the diet can impact their fermentation in the gut. For example, the amount of beta-glucans in a food source, their structure, and their solubility can affect how easily they can be fermented by gut bacteria.

2. Gut microbiota composition: The presence and abundance of different types of gut bacteria can influence the fermentation of beta-glucans. For instance, people with higher levels of Bifidobacterium and Lactobacillus in their gut are likely to have more efficient fermentation of beta-glucans, as these bacteria are known to be involved in this process.

3. Gut dysbiosis: Gut dysbiosis refers to an imbalance in gut microbiota composition, which can negatively affect beta-glucans fermentation. Various factors, such as the use of antibiotics, certain medical conditions, and a diet low in fiber, can cause dysbiosis. In cases of dysbiosis, there may be a reduction in the abundance of beneficial bacteria involved in the fermentation of beta-glucans, leading to decreased fermentation and the production of fewer SCFAs.

4. Other factors that can impact the fermentation of beta-glucans include age, genetics, and environmental factors such as stress. For instance, older adults tend to have a less diverse gut microbiota, which may affect the ability to ferment beta-glucans efficiently.

Therefore, the fermentation of beta-glucans in the gut is a complex process that is influenced by several factors, including diet, gut microbiota composition, gut dysbiosis, age, genetics, and environmental factors.

Gut microbiome modulation and digestive health

The gut microbiome is a complex ecosystem of microorganisms that is critical to human health, including digestive health. Modulating the gut microbiome through various interventions has positively impacted digestive health. Some ways to modulate the gut microbiome for improved digestive health include:

1. Probiotics: Probiotics are live microorganisms that provide health benefits when consumed in adequate amounts. Probiotics can help improve digestive health by restoring the balance of the gut microbiome, reducing inflammation, and enhancing the production of beneficial compounds like short-chain fatty acids (SCFAs).
2. Prebiotics: Prebiotics are indigestible fibers that serve as food for the beneficial bacteria in the gut. By promoting the growth of beneficial bacteria, prebiotics can improve digestive health by reducing inflammation, enhancing gut motility, and improving the absorption of nutrients.
3. Dietary fiber: Dietary fiber is an essential component of a healthy diet that can improve digestive health by promoting the growth of beneficial bacteria in the gut. Dietary fiber can also increase stool bulk, enhance gut motility, and reduce the risk of conditions like constipation, diverticulitis, and colorectal cancer.
4. Antibiotics: Antibiotics are medications that kill bacteria. While antibiotics are often necessary to treat bacterial infections, they can also disrupt the balance of the gut microbiome, leading to adverse effects on digestive health. Therefore, antibiotics should only be used when necessary, and probiotics and/or prebiotics may be recommended to restore the balance of the gut microbiome after antibiotic use.

5. Fecal microbiota transplantation (FMT): FMT is a procedure where fecal material from a healthy donor is transplanted into a person's gut with an unhealthy gut microbiome. FMT has shown promising results in treating conditions like Clostridioides difficile infection, inflammatory bowel disease, and irritable bowel syndrome.

In conclusion, modulating the gut microbiome through interventions like probiotics, prebiotics, dietary fiber, antibiotics, and FMT can improve digestive health by restoring the balance of the gut microbiome, reducing inflammation, enhancing gut motility, and improving the absorption of nutrients.

LEAKY GUT SYNDROME

Leaky Gut Syndrome, also known as increased intestinal permeability, is a condition in which the small intestine's lining becomes damaged, allowing substances that would usually be kept out to leak into the bloodstream.

The small intestine's lining acts as a barrier, allowing nutrients to pass into the bloodstream while keeping harmful substances out. When the lining becomes damaged, the barrier function is compromised, and substances that would usually be kept out can enter the bloodstream and cause inflammation and other health problems.

The leaked substances can include undigested food particles, toxins, and other harmful substances. This can lead to a wide range of symptoms and health problems, including digestive issues, autoimmune disorders, skin conditions, and even mental health issues.

Medical conditions associated with leaky gut

Leaky gut syndrome and gut microbiota dysbiosis have been linked to several medical conditions. Here are some examples:

1. Inflammatory bowel disease (IBD): IBD includes Crohn's disease and ulcerative colitis, characterized by chronic digestive tract inflammation. Both leaky gut syndrome and gut dysbiosis have been implicated in the development and progression of IBD.
2. Irritable bowel syndrome (IBS): IBS is a chronic digestive disorder characterized by abdominal pain, bloating, and changes in bowel habits. Studies have found that IBS patients often have abnormal gut microbiota and increased intestinal permeability.
3. Celiac disease: Celiac disease is an autoimmune disorder in which the immune system attacks the lining of the small intestine in response to gluten consumption. Leaky gut syndrome may play a role in the development of celiac disease, as increased intestinal permeability can allow gluten particles to enter the bloodstream and trigger an immune response.
4. Food allergies and sensitivities: Leaky gut syndrome has been linked to the development of food allergies and sensitivities, as it allows larger food particles to enter the bloodstream and trigger an immune response.
5. Obesity and metabolic syndrome: Studies have found that gut dysbiosis and increased intestinal permeability

may contribute to obesity and metabolic syndrome by altering the body's nutrient absorption and metabolic processes.

Overall, the exact mechanisms by which leaky gut syndrome and gut microbiota dysbiosis contribute to these medical conditions are still being investigated. However, it is clear that maintaining a healthy gut is important for overall health and may help prevent or manage certain medical conditions.

Symptoms of leaky gut

Leaky gut syndrome, also known as increased intestinal permeability, is a condition in which the small intestine's lining becomes damaged, allowing substances that would usually be kept out to leak into the bloodstream. This can lead to inflammation and a range of health problems, including digestive issues, autoimmune disorders, skin conditions, and hormonal imbalances.

Common symptoms of leaky gut include digestive issues, food sensitivities, skin problems, autoimmune conditions, fatigue, mood disorders, joint pain, headaches, and hormonal imbalances. However, the existence of leaky gut syndrome is still debated in the medical community, and more research is needed to understand its causes and effects fully.

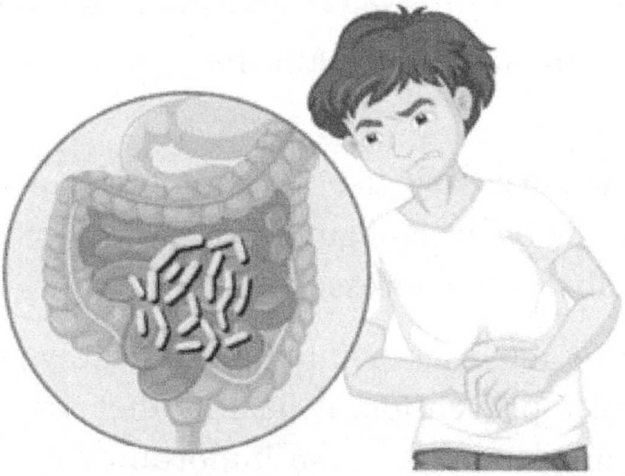

Obesity, leaky gut, and prevention

Growing evidence suggests that leaky gut syndrome may contribute to obesity and metabolic syndrome by altering nutrient absorption and metabolic processes in the body. Here are some ways to prevent a leaky gut and potentially reduce the risk of obesity:

1. Eat a healthy, balanced diet: A diet rich in fruits, vegetables, whole grains, lean protein, and healthy fats can help maintain gut health and reduce inflammation.
2. Avoid processed and high-sugar foods: These foods can promote inflammation and disrupt the balance of gut bacteria.
3. Consider taking probiotics: Probiotics are beneficial bacteria that can help restore the balance of gut bacteria and improve gut health.
4. Reduce stress: Chronic stress can increase inflammation in the body and contribute to a leaky gut. Strategies like exercise, meditation, and deep breathing can help reduce stress.

5. Get enough sleep: Poor sleep can disrupt gut health and increase inflammation. Aim for 7-8 hours of sleep per night.
6. Avoid unnecessary use of antibiotics: Antibiotics can disrupt the balance of gut bacteria, so avoid taking them unless absolutely necessary.

It's important to note that maintaining a healthy gut is just one aspect of obesity prevention. A healthy diet, regular exercise, and stress management are also important for maintaining a healthy weight. Consult with a healthcare provider to determine the best approach for you.

Causes of a leaky gut syndrome

The exact causes of the leaky gut syndrome are not fully understood, but several factors may contribute to its development. These include:

1. Poor diet: A diet high in processed foods, refined sugars, and unhealthy fats can promote inflammation in the gut and damage the intestinal lining.

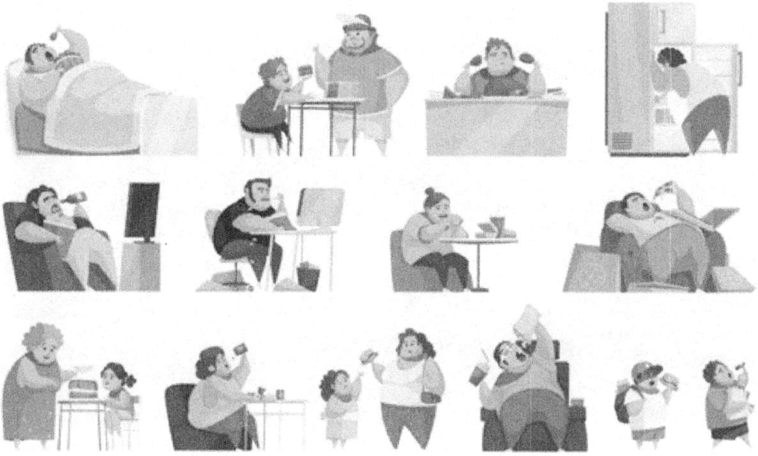

2. Chronic stress: Stress can increase inflammation in the body and disrupt the balance of gut bacteria.

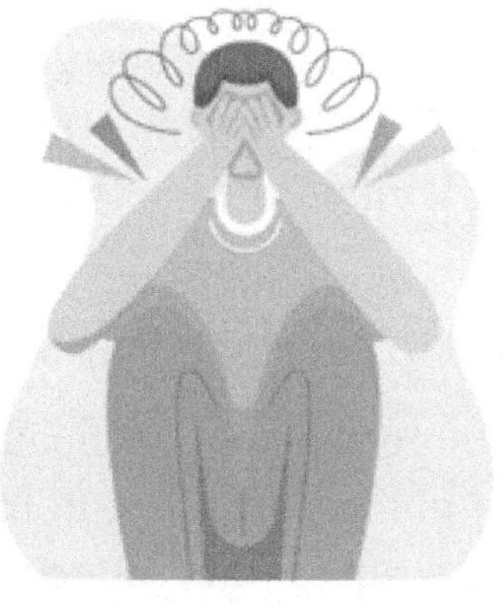

3. Overuse of antibiotics: Antibiotics can disrupt the balance of gut bacteria, which can lead to an overgrowth of harmful bacteria and damage to the intestinal lining.

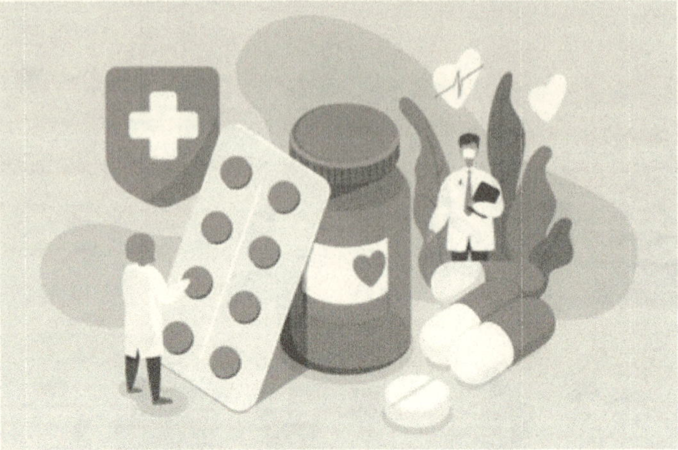

4. Environmental toxins: Exposure to toxins like pesticides, heavy metals, and pollution can damage the intestinal lining and promote inflammation.
5. Intestinal infections: Infections like SIBO (small intestinal bacterial overgrowth) and Candida overgrowth can damage the intestinal lining and promote inflammation.
6. Genetics: Some individuals may be genetically predisposed to developing the leaky gut syndrome.

It's important to note that not all health experts agree on the existence of leaky gut syndrome, and more research is needed to understand its causes and effects fully. However, many factors contributing to a leaky gut are also associated with poor gut health, so it's still essential to maintain a healthy gut.

Beta-glucan reduces the risk of leaking gut

Although research on the direct relationship between beta-glucan intake and leaky gut is limited, some studies have shown that beta-glucan can support gut health in various ways:

1. Prebiotic effect: Beta-glucan acts as a prebiotic, promoting the growth of beneficial gut bacteria, such as Lactobacillus and Bifidobacterium species. A healthy gut microbiome is essential for maintaining a strong intestinal barrier and preventing leaky gut.
2. Anti-inflammatory properties: Beta-glucan has been shown to exhibit anti-inflammatory effects, which can help reduce inflammation in the gut lining and protect the integrity of the intestinal barrier.
3. Enhancing gut barrier function: Some research suggests that beta-glucan may improve the gut barrier function by stimulating mucus production and increasing the expression of tight junction proteins, which are crucial for maintaining the integrity of the gut lining.
4. Immune modulation: Beta-glucan can modulate the immune system by activating immune cells, such as macrophages and neutrophils, and promoting the production of cytokines, which can help maintain a balanced immune response in the gut and prevent excessive inflammation.

It is important to consult with a healthcare professional before starting any new dietary supplement or making significant changes to your diet, especially if you have an existing medical condition.

Beta-glucan and short-chain fatty acids

Beta-glucan, as a type of soluble dietary fiber, can be fermented by the gut microbiota in the large intestine, producing short-chain fatty acids (SCFAs). SCFAs, primarily acetate, propionate, and butyrate, are known to have various health benefits. The relationship between beta-glucan intake, SCFA production, and health benefits is as follows:

1. Improved gut health: SCFAs, particularly butyrate, serve as the primary energy source for the colonocytes (cells lining the colon). This helps maintain the integrity of the gut barrier and promotes overall gut health. Moreover, SCFAs can lower the gut's pH, inhibiting the growth of harmful bacteria and supporting the development of beneficial bacteria, contributing to a healthy gut microbiome.
2. Anti-inflammatory effects: SCFAs have been shown to exhibit anti-inflammatory properties by modulating the immune system and inhibiting the production of pro-inflammatory cytokines. This can help reduce inflammation in various tissues, including the gut, which is particularly relevant for conditions like inflammatory bowel disease.
3. Enhanced glucose metabolism and insulin sensitivity: SCFAs, especially propionate, have been found to improve glucose metabolism and insulin sensitivity. Propionate can increase the production of the hormone glucagon-like peptide-1 (GLP-1), which stimulates insulin secretion and reduces blood sugar levels. Moreover, SCFAs can increase the uptake of glucose by muscle cells, contributing to better glycemic control.

4. Weight management and appetite regulation: SCFAs can help regulate appetite by stimulating the release of appetite-suppressing hormones like peptide YY (PYY) and GLP-1. Additionally, SCFAs can improve energy expenditure and fat oxidation, promoting weight management.

5. Cardiovascular health: SCFAs, particularly propionate, can help lower cholesterol levels by inhibiting cholesterol synthesis in the liver. This, in turn, can reduce the risk of developing cardiovascular diseases like atherosclerosis.

6. Cancer prevention: Butyrate has been shown to have anti-cancer properties, primarily by promoting apoptosis (cell death) in cancer cells and inhibiting cell proliferation. This is particularly relevant for colorectal cancer, as butyrate is produced in high concentrations in the colon.

In conclusion, consuming beta-glucan-rich foods can support the production of SCFAs by the gut microbiota, which in turn can have various health benefits. These include improved gut health, reduced inflammation, better glucose metabolism, weight management, cardiovascular health, and potentially cancer prevention. Therefore, incorporating beta-glucan-rich foods such as oats, barley, and certain mushrooms into a balanced diet can help promote overall health and well-being. However, consulting with a healthcare professional before significantly changing your diet is always a good idea.

Can IBD patients have a high-fiber or beta-glucan diet?

Inflammatory bowel disease (IBD) is a group of disorders that cause chronic inflammation in the gastrointestinal (GI) tract.

The two main types of IBD are Crohn's disease and ulcerative colitis. Diet plays a crucial role in managing IBD symptoms and preventing flare-ups. While fiber and beta-glucan have numerous health benefits, IBD patients must consider their needs and tolerance before making dietary changes.

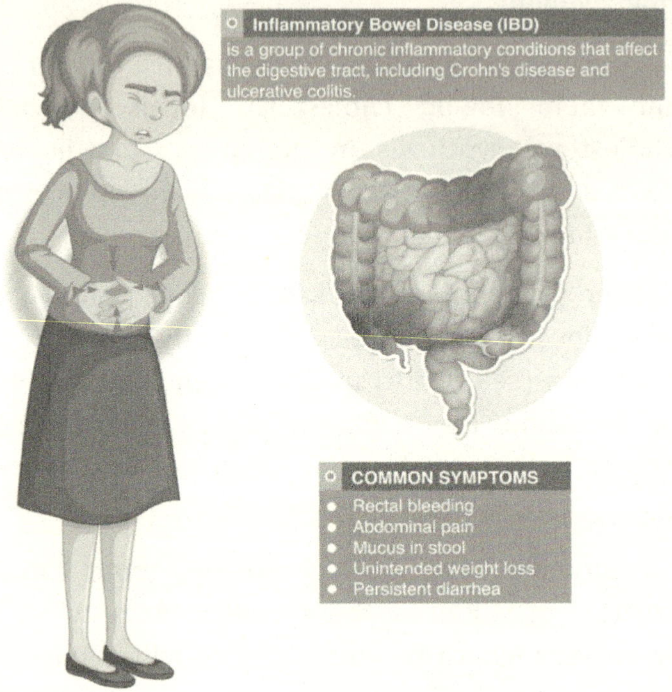

Generally, a high-fiber diet may benefit IBD patients during remission periods when inflammation is under control. In addition, fiber can help promote a healthy gut microbiome, maintain regular bowel movements, and reduce the risk of colorectal cancer, which is elevated in IBD patients.

However, a high-fiber diet may not be suitable for some IBD patients during active inflammation or flare-ups. This is because:

1. Mechanical irritation: Insoluble fiber found in foods like whole grains, fruits, and vegetables can add bulk to the stool and, in some cases, mechanically irritate the inflamed gut lining, potentially exacerbating IBD symptoms.
2. Increased gas production: Fermentation of soluble fiber, such as beta-glucan, by gut bacteria can lead to increased gas production, which may cause bloating, cramping, and abdominal discomfort in some IBD patients.

In the case of beta-glucan specifically, it is a soluble fiber that can help maintain gut health, support the immune system, and provide anti-inflammatory benefits. These properties could benefit IBD patients during remission, but caution should be exercised during flare-ups as fermentation of soluble fiber can still cause increased gas production and discomfort.

IBD patients must work closely with their healthcare providers or dietitians to develop a personalized dietary plan that considers their needs, tolerance, and disease status. For example, some IBD patients may tolerate moderate amounts of fiber or beta-glucan, while others may need to limit their intake during flare-ups and gradually reintroduce fiber as inflammation subsides.

In summary, IBD patients should be cautious when considering a high-fiber or beta-glucan diet, particularly during periods of active inflammation. It is essential to work with a healthcare professional to create a personalized dietary plan that takes into account individual needs, tolerance, and disease activity.

CHAPTER 8: HOW TO INCREASE YOUR BETA-GLUCAN INTAKE

Increasing your beta-glucan intake can have many health benefits, including reducing cholesterol levels, improving immune function, and regulating blood sugar levels. Good sources of beta-glucan include oats, barley, mushrooms, seaweed, and some types of yeast.

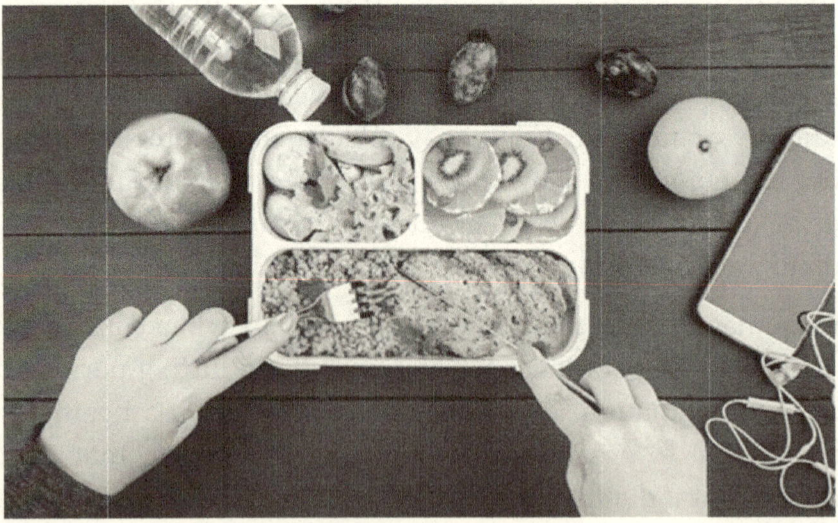

Incorporating these foods into your diet can be as simple as starting your day with a bowl of oatmeal, using barley in soups and salads, adding mushrooms to stir-fries or soups, snacking on whole grain crackers or granola bars, and considering a beta-glucan supplement if necessary. Additionally, drinking plenty of water is important to help absorb fiber-rich foods properly and keep you full and satisfied.

Food rich in beta-glucan

Beta-glucans are a type of soluble fiber found in certain foods that have been shown to improve metabolic health, reduce obesity, and lower the risk of developing metabolic syndrome.

Here is a list of six foods rich in beta-glucans, ranked from highest to lowest content:

1. Oats: Whole oats and oat bran are known for their high beta-glucan content, with about 2-8% of dry weight. Oats are also beneficial for maintaining a healthy weight and regulating blood sugar levels.
2. Barley: Hulled or pearled barley is an excellent source of beta-glucans. It contains about 2-8% beta-glucan content by dry weight, making it the richest source among these foods.
3. Whole grains: Wheat, rye, and sorghum are other sources of beta-glucans, though in lower amounts than barley and oats. Their content ranges between 0.5-2% by dry weight.
4. Mushrooms: Some varieties of mushrooms, such as shiitake, maitake, and reishi, contain beta-glucans. While the content is lower than that of grains, they can still contribute to a healthy diet.

5. Seaweed: Beta-glucans can be found in certain types of seaweed, including nori, wakame, and kelp. The content is much lower than in grains but can still provide some benefits.
6. Baker's yeast (Saccharomyces cerevisiae): While not commonly consumed as a food, baker's yeast is a source of beta-glucans. It can be found in nutritional supplements, and its consumption may have health benefits related to obesity and metabolic syndrome.

Remember, incorporating a variety of these beta-glucan-rich foods into your diet and maintaining a balanced and nutritious diet is essential for managing obesity and reducing the risk of metabolic syndrome.

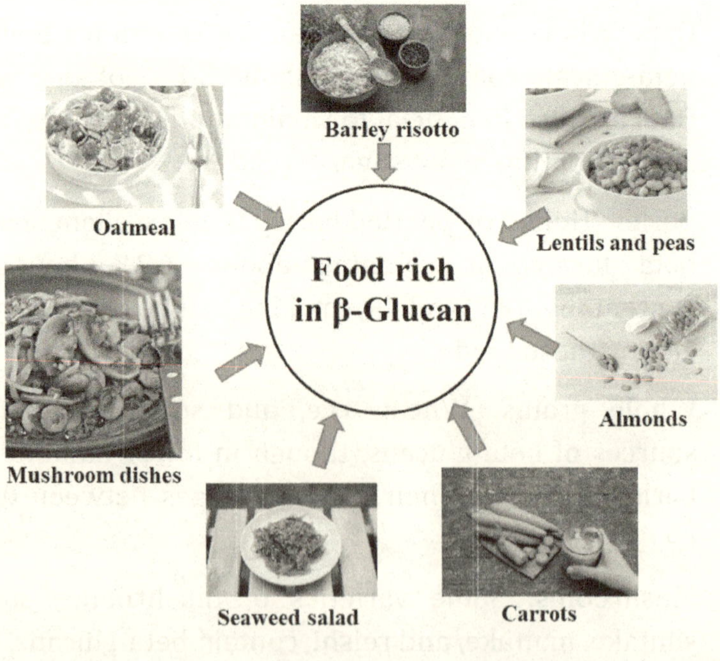

Practical tips

Incorporating beta-glucan-rich foods into your diet can be easy and enjoyable. Here are some practical tips to help you add these foods to your meals to manage obesity and metabolic syndrome:

1. Breakfast: Start your day with a bowl of oatmeal or oat bran cereal. Add fruits, nuts, and seeds for extra nutrients and flavor. You can also include barley flakes as an alternative or mix them with oats.
2. Baking: Use oat flour or barley flour in your baking recipes, like bread, muffins, pancakes, or cookies. You can replace a portion of the regular wheat flour with this beta-glucan-rich flour.
3. Grains: Include barley, whole wheat, or rye as a side dish or as part of your main meal. You can cook these grains like rice or use them in salads, soups, and stews.
4. Snacks: Opt for whole-grain crackers, rice cakes, or granola bars made with oats or barley for a beta-glucan-rich snack. Be mindful of added sugars and fats in store-bought products.
5. Mushroom dishes: Incorporate beta-glucan-rich mushrooms like shiitake, maitake, or reishi into your meals by adding them to stir-fries, soups, or pasta dishes.
6. Seaweed: Add seaweed like nori, wakame, or kelp to your diet by including them in sushi rolls, salads, or soups.
7. Supplements: If you find it challenging to include enough beta-glucan-rich foods in your diet, consider taking a supplement containing beta-glucans derived

from yeast or mushrooms. Consult your healthcare provider before starting any supplements.

8. Mindful eating: Pay attention to portion sizes and avoid overeating, even with healthy foods. Eating slowly and savoring each bite can help with portion control.
9. Balanced diet: Remember to maintain a well-balanced diet that includes a variety of fruits, vegetables, lean proteins, and healthy fats, along with beta-glucan-rich foods.
10. Physical activity: Incorporate regular physical activity into your lifestyle to complement your dietary efforts in managing obesity and metabolic syndrome. Aim for at least 150 minutes of moderate-intensity aerobic exercise or 75 minutes of vigorous-intensity aerobic exercise per week, along with muscle-strengthening activities on two or more days per week.

By following these tips and adjusting your lifestyle, you can effectively incorporate beta-glucan-rich foods into your diet and improve your overall health.

Supplements and fortified foods

Supplements and fortified foods can also serve as sources of beta-glucans for individuals looking to manage obesity and metabolic disorders. These options can be beneficial, especially for those who struggle to consume adequate amounts of beta-glucan-rich foods in their daily diet. However, consulting with a healthcare provider before starting any supplements is essential.

1. Beta-glucan supplements: Available in capsules, tablets, or powders, these supplements are typically derived from yeast (Saccharomyces cerevisiae) or mushrooms (like shiitake, maitake, and reishi). They can provide a concentrated source of beta-glucans and help improve metabolic health. Be sure to choose a reputable brand and follow the recommended dosage guidelines.
2. Fortified foods: Some food products, like cereals, granola bars, and beverages, are fortified with beta-glucans. These products can be a convenient way to increase your beta-glucan intake. However, be cautious of added sugars, fats, and artificial ingredients in some fortified products, which may negate the health benefits.

When considering supplements and fortified foods as sources of beta-glucans, keep the following in mind:

- Consult your healthcare provider before starting any supplements, especially if you have any pre-existing medical conditions or are taking medications, as there may be potential interactions.
- Maintaining a balanced and nutritious diet, including whole foods like fruits, vegetables, whole grains, lean proteins, and healthy fats, is essential. Supplements and fortified foods should complement, not replace, a healthy diet.
- Monitor your progress and adjust your intake as needed. Regularly consult with your healthcare provider to ensure the beta-glucan supplements or fortified foods are effectively helping manage your obesity and metabolic disorders.

- Incorporate regular physical activity into your lifestyle to further support your dietary efforts in managing obesity and metabolic syndrome.

Combining supplements and fortified foods with a balanced diet and an active lifestyle can effectively manage obesity and metabolic disorders and improve your overall health.

Fortified foods with beta-glucan

Here are some examples of fortified foods with beta-glucan that are available in Australia:

1. Uncle Tobys Oats: Uncle Tobys offers a range of oat-based products that are high in beta-glucan, including traditional oats, quick oats, and instant oats.
2. Sanitarium Weet-Bix: Weet-Bix is a popular breakfast cereal in Australia that is made from whole grains, including wheat and barley, and is high in beta-glucan.
3. Vogel's Soy & Linseed Bread: This bread is fortified with oat bran, which is a good source of beta-glucan. It's great for those who prefer bread over cereals and other breakfast options.
4. Freedom Foods Barley+ Muesli: This muesli is made from a blend of whole grains, including barley, and is high in beta-glucan. It's a great option for those who prefer a cereal-like breakfast.
5. Kellogg's Nutri-Grain: Nutri-Grain is a popular breakfast cereal in Australia fortified with oat fiber, a good source of beta-glucan.

Several fortified food products containing beta-glucans are available in the USA. Keep in mind that product availability may vary by location and store. Some examples of beta-glucan-fortified foods include:

1. Cereals:
    - Cheerios Oat Crunch
    - Nature's Path SmartBran
    - General Mills' Heart to Heart Oat Cereal
    - Kellogg's All-Bran Original Cereal
2. Granola Bars:
    - Nature Valley Oats 'n Honey Crunchy Granola Bars
    - Quaker Chewy Oat Granola Bars
    - Kind Oats & Honey with Toasted Coconut
3. Beverages:
    - Quaker Oat Beverage
    - Simpli Instant Oat Shake
    - Oatly Oat Milk
4. Breads:
    - Dave's Killer Bread - Good Seed Bread
    - Rudi's Organic Bakery - 7 Grain with Flax
5. Meal replacement shakes and protein powders:
    - Garden of Life Raw Organic Meal Replacement
    - Vega One All-in-One Shake

Check the nutrition labels for beta-glucan content and be aware of added sugars, fats, and artificial ingredients in some fortified products. As always, it's essential to maintain a balanced and nutritious diet, including whole foods like fruits, vegetables, whole grains, lean proteins, and healthy fats. Supplements and fortified foods should complement, not replace, a healthy diet.

CHAPTER 9: RECIPES AND MEAL PLANS

There are several reasons why you may want to develop recipes and meal plans for a beta-glucan-rich diet:

There are several reasons why you may want to develop recipes and meal plans for a beta-glucan-rich diet:

1. Heart health: Beta-glucans can help lower cholesterol levels, which is essential for heart health. A diet rich in beta-glucans from sources such as oats, barley, and legumes can help reduce the risk of heart disease.

2. Immune function: Beta-glucans can help stimulate the immune system, making it more effective in fighting off infections and diseases. A diet rich in beta-glucans from sources such as mushrooms and oats can help support immune function.

3. Gut health: Beta-glucans are a type of prebiotic fiber that can feed the good bacteria in your gut, promoting a healthy gut microbiome. A diet rich in beta-glucans from sources such as oats, barley, and legumes can help support gut health.

4. Weight management: Beta-glucans can help you feel full and satisfied, which can help with weight management.

A diet rich in beta-glucans from sources such as oats, barley, and legumes can help you feel full and satisfied for longer periods of time.

5. Diabetes management: Beta-glucans can help regulate blood sugar levels, making them beneficial for people with diabetes. A diet rich in beta-glucans from sources such as oats, barley, and legumes can help with diabetes management.

Developing recipes and meal plans that are rich in beta-glucans can help you incorporate these important nutrients into your diet in a tasty and satisfying way. It can also help you reap the many health benefits associated with beta-glucans.

Delicious Recipes Rich in Beta-Glucan

Oatmeal and banana pancakes

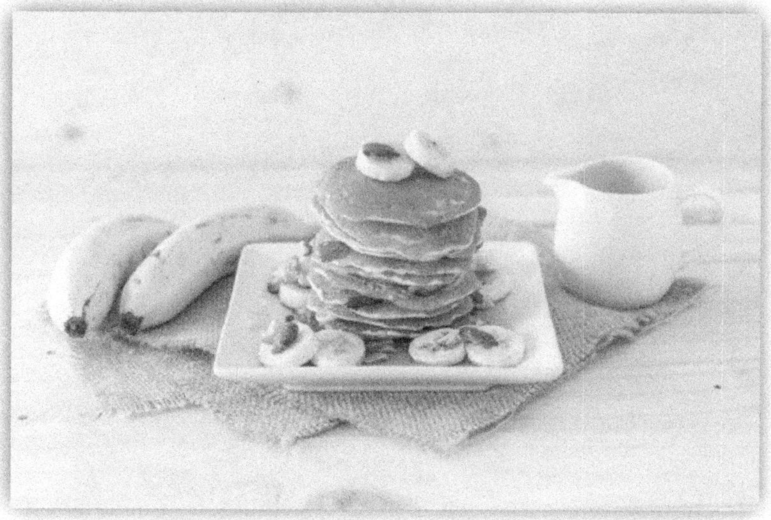

Receips: 1 cup of oats, 1/2 cup of flour, 1 tsp of baking powder, 1/2 tsp of baking soda, 1/4 tsp of salt, 1 banana, mashed, 1 cup of milk, 2 eggs, 1 tsp of vanilla extract

Cook: In a large bowl, mix together the dry ingredients. In a separate bowl, mash the banana and then add the milk, eggs, and vanilla extract. Mix the wet ingredients into the dry ingredients until well combined. Heat a non-stick skillet over medium heat and drop 1/4 cup of batter for each pancake. Cook until the edges are set, and bubbles form on the surface, then flip and cook for an additional 1-2 minutes.

Mushroom and barley risotto

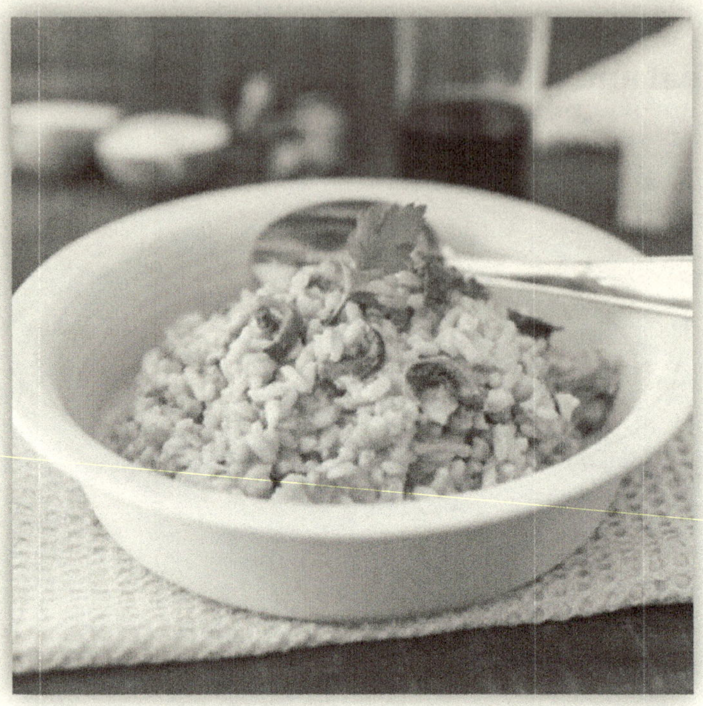

Receips: 2 tbsp of olive oil, 1 onion, chopped, 3 cloves of garlic, minced, 1 cup of barley, 4 cups of vegetable broth, 1/2 cup of white wine, 200g of mushrooms, sliced, 1/2 cup of grated cheese, Salt and pepper, to taste

Cook: In a large pot, heat the olive oil over medium heat. Add the onion and garlic and sauté until softened, about 5 minutes. Add the barley and stir to coat with the oil. Pour in the vegetable broth and white wine and bring to a simmer. Cook until the barley is tender and the liquid is absorbed, about 45 minutes. In a separate skillet, sauté the mushrooms until browned and tender. Stir the mushrooms and Parmesan cheese into the barley mixture and season with salt and pepper.

Lentil and carrot soup

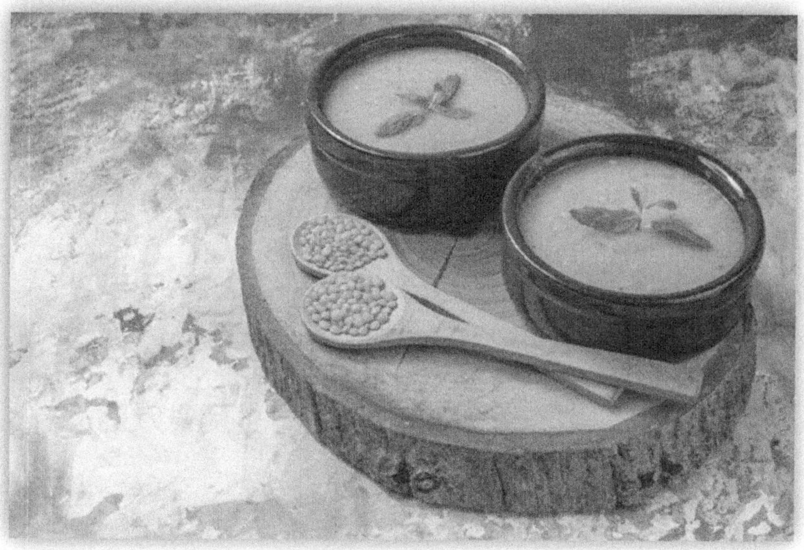

Receips: 1 onion, chopped, 2 cloves of garlic, minced, 4 carrots, peeled and chopped, 1 cup of red lentils, 4 cups of vegetable broth, 1 tsp of ground cumin, 1 tsp of ground coriander, Salt and pepper, to taste

Cook: In a large pot, heat a drizzle of oil over medium heat. Add the onion and garlic and sauté until softened, about 5 minutes. Add the carrots and continue to sauté until they start to soften, another 5-7 minutes. Stir in the lentils, vegetable broth, cumin, and coriander. Bring to a simmer and cook until the lentils are tender, about 20-25 minutes. Season with salt and pepper to taste.

These suggested recipes are not only delicious, but they're also a great way to incorporate beta-glucan-rich foods into your diet.

MEAL PLANS TO INCREASE BETA-GLUCAN INTAKE

For obesity and metabolic syndrome

A three-day meal plan with high beta-glucan for obesity and metabolic syndrome

Beta-glucan is a dietary fiber in foods like oats, barley, and mushrooms. It has been shown to have beneficial effects on obesity and metabolic syndrome by improving cholesterol levels, reducing blood sugar, and promoting a feeling of fullness. Here is a three-day meal plan that includes foods high in beta-glucan:

Day 1:

- Breakfast: Overnight oats with almond milk, chia seeds, and berries; Green smoothie with spinach, kale, and a small banana
- Lunch: Lentil and barley soup with mixed vegetables; Side salad with mixed greens, cherry tomatoes, and a light vinaigrette
- Dinner: Grilled salmon with barley and roasted vegetable pilaf; Steamed broccoli
- Snack: Sliced apple with almond butter
    -

Day 2:

- Breakfast: Oat bran pancake with fresh berries and a dollop of Greek yogurt; Herbal tea or black coffee

- Lunch: Chickpea and barley salad with cucumber, bell peppers, and a lemon-tahini dressing; Sliced avocado with a sprinkle of sea salt
- Dinner: Mushroom stroganoff with whole-grain pasta (use a variety of mushrooms high in beta-glucan, such as shiitake or maitake); Steamed green beans
- Snack: Greek yogurt with a tablespoon of honey and a sprinkle of ground flaxseeds

Day 3:

- Breakfast: Chia pudding with almond milk, topped with fresh berries and a drizzle of honey; Green tea
- Lunch: Oat bran pita stuffed with grilled chicken, mixed greens, and tzatziki sauce; Sliced carrots and hummus
- Dinner: Vegetable stir-fry with tofu, mixed vegetables, and shiitake mushrooms, served over brown rice; Steamed edamame
- Snack: A small bowl of air-popped popcorn with a sprinkle of nutritional yeast

Remember to drink plenty of water throughout the day, as beta-glucan absorbs water and can help you feel fuller. Combining these meals with regular physical activity and a balanced diet is essential for the best results in managing obesity and metabolic syndrome. Always consult your doctor or a nutritionist before significantly changing your diet.

For heart health and hypertension

Beta-glucan is a type of soluble fiber found in certain foods like oats, barley, and certain mushrooms. Including beta-glucan-rich foods in your diet can help improve heart health and lower hypertension and cholesterol levels. Here is a three-day meal plan with high beta-glucan content for you:

Day 1:

- Breakfast: Overnight oats with berries and chia seeds; A glass of freshly squeezed orange juice
- Lunch: Barley and vegetable salad with lemon-tahini dressing; Whole grain bread; 1 apple
- Dinner: Oat-crusted baked salmon with steamed vegetables; Quinoa and mushroom pilaf
- Snack: 1 small handful of almonds

Day 2:

- Breakfast: Oat and banana smoothie with almond milk, flaxseeds, and honey; A bowl of mixed fruit salad
- Lunch: Mushroom barley soup with whole grain bread; Baby spinach and avocado salad
- Dinner: Oat and herb-stuffed bell peppers; Steamed green beans; Roasted sweet potatoes
- Snack: Baby carrots and hummus

Day 3:

- Breakfast: Oat and quinoa porridge with dried fruits, nuts, and a drizzle of maple syrup; A cup of green tea
- Lunch: Barley, chickpea, and roasted vegetable salad with lemon-olive oil dressing; A pear
- Dinner: Oat-breaded chicken breast with a mixed green salad; Baked zucchini and tomato casserole
- Snack: Greek yogurt with honey and walnuts

Please note that these meal plans are only suggestions. It is essential to consult with a registered dietitian or nutritionist to create a personalized meal plan that meets your specific needs and health goals.

For type 2 diabetes

Here's a simple three-day meal plan with high beta-glucan content, suitable for individuals with Type 2 diabetes. This meal plan focuses on incorporating whole grains, legumes, fruits, and vegetables that are rich in beta-glucan, which has been shown to help control blood sugar levels.

Day 1:

- Breakfast: Overnight oats: 1/2 cup rolled oats, 1 tablespoon chia seeds, 1 cup unsweetened almond milk, 1/4 cup chopped almonds, and 1/4 cup berries. Mix ingredients and refrigerate overnight.
- Lunch: Lentil salad: 1 cup cooked lentils, 1/4 cup chopped red bell pepper, 1/4 cup chopped cucumber, 1/4 cup chopped red onion, 1 tablespoon olive oil, 2 tablespoons lemon juice, salt, and pepper to taste. Mix ingredients and serve chilled.
- Dinner: Barley and vegetable stir-fry: 1 cup cooked barley, 1 cup mixed vegetables (broccoli, carrots, bell peppers), 1/2 cup cubed tofu, 2 tablespoons low-sodium soy sauce, and 1 tablespoon sesame oil. Stir-fry vegetables and tofu in sesame oil, then mix in cooked barley and soy sauce.

Day 2:

- Breakfast: Barley porridge: 1/2 cup cooked pearled barley, 1/4 cup diced apple, 1 tablespoon of walnuts, 1 tablespoon of honey, and a pinch of cinnamon. Warm the barley and mix in the remaining ingredients.
- Lunch: Chickpea and quinoa salad: 1/2 cup cooked quinoa, 1/2 cup cooked chickpeas, 1/2 cup chopped cherry tomatoes, 1/2 cup chopped cucumber, 1/4 cup chopped red onion, 1 tablespoon olive oil, 2 tablespoons lemon juice, salt, and pepper to taste. Mix ingredients and serve chilled.
- Dinner: Mushroom barley soup: 1 cup cooked barley, 1 cup sliced mushrooms, 1/2 cup chopped onions, 1/2 cup chopped carrots, 1/2 cup chopped celery, 4 cups low-sodium vegetable broth, and 1 tablespoon olive oil. Sauté vegetables in olive oil, then add broth and cooked barley. Simmer until vegetables are tender.

Day 3:

- Breakfast: Oat bran cereal: 1/2 cup oat bran, 1 cup unsweetened almond milk, 1 tablespoon ground flaxseed, 1/4 cup berries, and a pinch of cinnamon. Cook oat bran with almond milk and top with flaxseed, berries, and cinnamon.
- Lunch: Black bean and barley wrap: 1/2 cup cooked barley, 1/2 cup cooked black beans, 1/4 cup chopped red bell pepper, 1/4 cup chopped avocado, 1/4 cup salsa, 1 whole-grain tortilla. Mix barley, black beans, bell pepper, and avocado, then place the mixture in the tortilla and top with salsa.
- Dinner: Whole grain pasta with mushrooms and peas: 1 cup cooked whole grain pasta, 1 cup sliced mushrooms, 1/2 cup peas, 1/4 cup grated Parmesan cheese, 1 tablespoon olive oil, salt, and pepper to taste. Sauté mushrooms and peas in

olive oil, then mix with cooked pasta and top with Parmesan cheese.

Remember to consult with your healthcare provider or a registered dietitian before making any significant changes to your diet, as individual needs may vary.

For individuals experiencing constipation

Here's a simple one-day meal plan high in beta-glucan for individuals experiencing constipation. Beta-glucan is a soluble fiber found in oats, barley, and some mushrooms, which can help improve bowel movements and support gut health. Always consult with a healthcare professional before making any significant changes to your diet.

- Breakfast: Overnight oats: Mix 1/2 cup of rolled oats, 1 cup of unsweetened almond milk, 1 tablespoon of chia seeds, and 1 teaspoon of honey or maple syrup. Store it in the refrigerator overnight. Add a handful of berries, chopped nuts, and a sprinkle of ground flaxseed in the morning.
- Morning Snack: A small apple or pear with the skin on (for added fiber) and a tablespoon of natural almond or peanut butter.
- Lunch: Barley salad: Toss 1 cup of cooked barley with diced cucumber, cherry tomatoes, chopped bell peppers, and red onion. Add a handful of chopped fresh parsley, a drizzle of olive oil, a squeeze of lemon juice, salt, and pepper to taste.
- Afternoon Snack: Greek yogurt with a tablespoon of honey and a handful of raspberries or blueberries.
- Dinner: Mushroom barley soup: Cook 1 cup of barley according to package instructions. In a separate pot, sauté sliced onions, carrots, and celery in olive oil. Add sliced

mushrooms, vegetable broth, cooked barley, and seasoning (thyme, rosemary, salt, and pepper). Let it simmer for 30 minutes.

- Evening Snack: 2-3 oat bran crackers with a thin layer of hummus or avocado.

Remember to drink plenty of water throughout the day to help promote healthy bowel movements. It's also important to introduce high-fiber foods gradually to avoid potential digestive discomfort or gas.

Museli bar for satiety control

Making a muesli bar high in beta-glucan can help increase satiety and provide a great source of fiber. Here's a simple recipe for homemade muesli bars that are rich in beta-glucan from oats and barley flakes:

Ingredients:

1/2 cups rolled oats (rich in beta-glucan); 1/2 cup barley flakes (rich in beta-glucan); 1/2 cup chopped nuts (e.g., almonds, walnuts, or pecans); 1/4 cup dried fruit (e.g., raisins, cranberries, or chopped dates); 1/4 cup unsweetened shredded coconut; 2 tablespoons chia seeds or ground flaxseeds; 1/2 teaspoon cinnamon; 1/4 teaspoon salt; 1/3 cup honey or maple syrup; 1/4 cup natural peanut or almond butter; 1 teaspoon vanilla extract

Instructions:

1. Preheat your oven to 350°F (175°C) and line an 8x8-inch baking dish with parchment paper, allowing the paper to overhang the sides for easy removal.
2. Combine the rolled oats, barley flakes, chopped nuts, dried fruit, shredded coconut, chia or flaxseeds, cinnamon, and salt in a large mixing bowl. Mix well.
3. In a small saucepan, gently heat the honey or maple syrup and nut butter over low heat, stirring until the mixture is smooth and well-combined. Remove from heat and stir in the vanilla extract.
4. Pour the wet mixture over the dry ingredients, and mix well, ensuring that all the dry ingredients are coated.
5. Transfer the mixture to the prepared baking dish, and press it firmly into an even layer using a spatula or your hands.
6. Bake for 20-25 minutes or until the edges are golden brown. Remove from the oven and allow the muesli bars to cool completely in the baking dish.
7. Once cooled, use the parchment paper to lift the muesli bars out of the dish. Cut into bars or squares using a sharp knife.
8. Store the muesli bars in an airtight container at room temperature for up to one week or in the refrigerator for up to two weeks.

These muesli bars are high in beta-glucan and provide a good balance of healthy fats, protein, and carbohydrates to keep you full and satisfied.

Museli bar to boost immunity

Beta-1,3/1,6-glucan is a specific type of beta-glucan found in the cell walls of baker's yeast (Saccharomyces cerevisiae), medicinal mushrooms like shiitake and maitake, and some seaweeds. This type of beta-glucan is known for its immune-boosting properties. To make a muesli bar containing high beta-1,3/1,6-glucan, you can use a powdered supplement, which can be easily added to recipes. Here's a simple recipe:

Ingredients:

2 cups rolled oats; 1/2 cup chopped nuts (e.g., almonds, walnuts, or cashews);1/2 cup dried fruit (e.g., raisins, cranberries, or chopped dates); 1/4 cup unsweetened shredded coconut; 1/4 cup ground flaxseed; 1/4 cup honey or maple syrup; 1/4 cup almond or peanut butter; 1 teaspoon vanilla extract; 1/4 teaspoon salt; 1/2 teaspoon cinnamon; 2 tablespoons beta-1,3/1,6-glucan powder (from a reputable supplement brand)

Instructions:

1. Preheat your oven to 350°F (180°C). Line an 8-inch square baking dish with parchment paper, leaving some overhang for easy removal.
2. Combine rolled oats, chopped nuts, dried fruit, shredded coconut, and ground flaxseed in a large mixing bowl.
3. Combine honey or maple syrup, almond or peanut butter, vanilla extract, salt, and cinnamon in a small saucepan over low heat. Stir until smooth and well combined.

4. Remove the saucepan from heat and carefully mix in the beta-1,3/1,6-glucan powder until fully incorporated.
5. Pour the wet mixture over the dry ingredients and mix well, ensuring that all ingredients are evenly coated.
6. Transfer the mixture to the prepared baking dish, pressing it down firmly and evenly.
7. Bake for 20-25 minutes or until the edges are golden brown. Allow the muesli bars to cool completely in the baking dish before lifting the parchment paper and placing them on a cutting board. Cut into bars or squares.
8. Store the muesli bars in an airtight container at room temperature for up to one week, or refrigerate for longer shelf life.

Note: Always consult a healthcare professional before adding supplements to your diet, especially if you have a medical condition or are taking medications.

Tips for meal planning and preparation

Here are some tips for meal planning and preparation:

1. Plan ahead: Take some time to plan out your meals for the week. Make a grocery list of the ingredients you'll need, and stick to it when shopping.
2. Prep ahead: Prepping your meals ahead of time can save you a lot of time during the week. You can chop vegetables, cook grains and proteins, and even portion your weekly meals.
3. Use a slow cooker or pressure cooker: Slow and pressure cookers are great tools for meal preparation. You can cook

large batches of food simultaneously, requiring minimal effort.

4. Keep it simple: Don't feel like you need to make elaborate meals every night. Simple meals like grilled chicken with roasted vegetables or a stir-fry with brown rice and mixed vegetables can be delicious and nutritious.
5. Batch cook: Cooking large batches of food at once can save you time and money. You can portion out your meals for the week and freeze them for later.
6. Get creative: Don't be afraid to experiment with new ingredients and flavors. Try new recipes, and don't be afraid to make substitutions based on your personal preferences or dietary restrictions.
7. Make it enjoyable: Meal planning and preparation can be an enjoyable process. Put on some music, involve your family or friends, and enjoy the process of creating delicious and nutritious meals.

CHAPTER 10: WHO CAN NOT HAVE HIGH FIBER INTAKE?

Who should not take a high-fiber diet?

A high-fiber diet is generally beneficial for most people, as it promotes healthy digestion, regulates blood sugar levels, and aids in maintaining a healthy weight. However, in certain situations, a high-fiber diet may not be appropriate or should be adjusted under medical supervision. Some of these situations include:

1. Individuals with gastrointestinal disorders: People with conditions such as Irritable Bowel Syndrome (IBS), Inflammatory Bowel Disease (IBD), or diverticulitis may need to limit or modify their fiber intake. A high-fiber diet may exacerbate symptoms like abdominal pain, bloating, and gas in some individuals.

2. Bowel obstruction: A high-fiber diet is not recommended for those with a partial or complete bowel obstruction, as it may worsen the situation. In such cases, a low-fiber or liquid diet is typically recommended.

3. Difficulty swallowing or chewing: People who have difficulty swallowing or chewing may have trouble consuming high-fiber foods like whole grains, fruits, and

vegetables. They may need to adjust their diet to include softer, more easily consumed sources of fiber.

4. Post-surgery or post-procedure recovery: After certain gastrointestinal surgeries or procedures, patients may be advised to follow a low-fiber diet temporarily to allow the digestive system to heal and recover.
5. Gastroparesis: This is a condition in which the stomach is slow to empty, and it may require a low-fiber diet, as fiber can slow down digestion even more.
6. Recent acute diarrhea or vomiting: In cases of acute diarrhea or vomiting, a low-fiber, bland diet is usually recommended temporarily to help the digestive system recover.
7. Individuals with kidney disease: Some people with kidney disease may need to limit their phosphorus intake, which may require limiting certain high-fiber foods, such as beans and whole grains.

It's important to consult with a healthcare professional or a registered dietitian before making any significant changes to your diet, especially if you have an existing medical condition or are taking medications. They can provide personalized advice based on your unique needs and health status.

Who can not have a high beta-glucan diet?

While beta-glucans are generally considered safe for consumption, some individuals may need to limit their intake or avoid a high beta-glucan diet altogether. These include:

1. People with celiac disease: Beta-glucans are found in some gluten-containing grains, such as barley, which is not

suitable for people with celiac disease. In these cases, alternative sources of beta-glucans, such as oats or mushrooms, can be consumed.

2. People with a yeast allergy: Beta-glucans are also found in yeast, and those with a yeast allergy should avoid consuming beta-glucans from yeast sources.
3. People taking certain medications: Beta-glucans can interact with certain medications, such as immunosuppressants and blood thinners. Therefore, individuals taking these medications should talk to their healthcare provider before increasing their beta-glucan intake.
4. Infants: While breast milk naturally contains beta-glucans, there is currently not enough evidence to support giving beta-glucan supplements to infants.
5. Those with gastrointestinal issues: As mentioned earlier, a high-fiber diet that includes beta-glucans may not be suitable for people with some gastrointestinal problems, such as inflammatory bowel disease. These individuals should work with a healthcare provider or registered dietitian to determine the best dietary approach for their needs.

It is always essential to consult with a healthcare provider before making any significant changes to your diet, especially if you have any underlying medical conditions or are taking medications.

CHAPTER 11: CONCLUSION AND RECOMMENDATIONS

Here is a summary of key points about beta-glucan dietary fiber and its benefits for obesity:

1. Beta-glucan is a soluble fiber found in oats, barley, mushrooms, and other foods.
2. Beta-glucan can help with weight loss by promoting satiety and reducing appetite, which may reduce overall calorie intake.
3. Beta-glucan can also improve blood sugar control, benefiting those with obesity and type 2 diabetes.
4. Consuming beta-glucan can improve lipid profile, such as reduced LDL cholesterol levels, which is vital for reducing the risk of cardiovascular disease.
5. To increase beta-glucan intake, include foods such as oats, barley, and mushrooms in your diet. You can also supplement with beta-glucan or consume fortified foods.
6. When incorporating beta-glucan-rich foods into your diet, it's crucial also to drink plenty of water to help the fiber do its job and prevent constipation.
7. Meal planning and preparation can help ensure you are getting enough beta-glucan in your diet while enjoying delicious and nutritious meals.

Beta-glucan is a beneficial dietary fiber that can help with weight loss and improve overall health, especially when combined with a healthy diet and lifestyle.

Practical tips

Incorporating beta-glucan into your diet and improving overall health can be achieved through a combination of practical tips, resources, and commitment. Here are some suggestions to help you get started:

1. Educate yourself: Learn about beta-glucan-rich foods, their health benefits, and how they can help manage obesity and metabolic disorders. Reputable sources like the American Heart Association, the Academy of Nutrition and Dietetics, or the World Health Organization can provide evidence-based information.
2. Plan your meals: Create a weekly meal plan that includes a variety of beta-glucan-rich foods, ensuring that you get adequate intake from different sources. Planning can help you avoid last-minute, unhealthy food choices.
3. Find recipes: Look for recipes incorporating beta-glucan-rich foods in creative and tasty ways. Websites like EatingWell, Allrecipes, and Food Network offer numerous recipes to help you create delicious and nutritious meals.
4. Shop smart: Make a shopping list based on your meal plan and stick to it. Choose whole, unprocessed foods and look for beta-glucan-fortified products with minimal added sugars and artificial ingredients.

5. Balanced diet: Along with beta-glucan-rich foods, ensure your diet includes a variety of fruits, vegetables, lean proteins, and healthy fats to maintain overall health.
6. Portion control: Be mindful of portion sizes, even with healthy foods. Using smaller plates, eating slowly, and listening to your body's hunger and fullness cues can help with portion control.
7. Cook at home: Preparing meals at home allows you to control the ingredients and cooking methods, making it easier to incorporate beta-glucan-rich foods into your diet.
8. Stay hydrated: Drink plenty of water throughout the day to support digestion and overall health.
9. Get active: Engage in regular physical activity to support your dietary efforts in managing obesity and metabolic syndrome. Aim for at least 150 minutes of moderate-intensity aerobic exercise or 75 minutes of vigorous-intensity aerobic exercise per week, along with muscle-strengthening activities on two or more days per week.
10. Seek support: Connect with a registered dietitian, nutritionist, or healthcare professional for personalized advice and guidance on incorporating beta-glucans into your diet and improving your overall health.

By following these tips and making use of available resources, you can successfully incorporate beta-glucan into your diet and achieve better overall health. Remember that consistency and commitment are key to reaching your health goals.

Future research directions

Beta-glucans have shown promising health benefits, but much remains to learn. Future directions for research on beta-glucans may include the following:

1. Mechanisms of action: Further investigation into the molecular mechanisms by which beta-glucans exert their health benefits, such as immune modulation, cholesterol-lowering effects, and blood sugar regulation.
2. Optimal dosage and formulation: Determining the optimal dosage, formulation, and type of beta-glucan (e.g., from oats, barley, yeast, or mushrooms) for specific health outcomes, as well as identifying potential synergistic effects with other nutrients or bioactive compounds.
3. Individual variability: Examining the influence of genetics, age, sex, and lifestyle factors on the effectiveness of beta-glucans, which could help tailor personalized dietary recommendations.
4. Long-term effects: Conducting long-term, large-scale studies to assess the sustained benefits of beta-glucan consumption on chronic diseases, such as cardiovascular disease, diabetes, and obesity.
5. Gut microbiota: Investigating the impact of beta-glucans on gut microbiota composition and function, which could reveal additional health benefits related to immune function, metabolism, and inflammation.
6. Food processing and bioavailability: Studying the effects of food processing and cooking methods on the bioavailability and functionality of beta-glucans to

optimize their health benefits in the context of real-world dietary practices.

7. Food applications: Developing novel food products and functional ingredients fortified with beta-glucans to increase their accessibility and promote their health benefits to a wider population.
8. Immune function and infection: Exploring the potential role of beta-glucans in enhancing immune function and reducing the risk or severity of infections, including viral respiratory infections and potential applications in the context of emerging infectious diseases.
9. Cancer research: Investigating the potential benefits of beta-glucans in cancer prevention and treatment, particularly their effects on immune function, inflammation, and tumor growth.
10. Neurological and mental health: Examining the potential impact of beta-glucans on brain function, cognitive health, and mental well-being, as well as their potential role in preventing or managing neurodegenerative diseases.

By addressing these research areas, scientists can deepen our understanding of the health benefits of beta-glucans and provide more comprehensive dietary recommendations for the prevention and management of various health conditions.

The future directions for public health

As research on beta-glucans continues to demonstrate their potential health benefits, public health initiatives can emphasize their importance for managing obesity, metabolic disorders, and other health conditions. Some future directions for public health initiatives focusing on beta-glucans might include:

1. Educational campaigns: Raise public awareness of the health benefits of beta-glucans through educational campaigns in schools, workplaces, and community centers, emphasizing the importance of consuming beta-glucan-rich foods.
2. Food labeling: Encourage food manufacturers to clearly label beta-glucan content on packaging to help consumers make informed choices and easily identify beta-glucan-rich products.
3. Accessibility and affordability: Work with government agencies, non-governmental organizations, and the food industry to increase the accessibility and affordability of beta-glucan-rich foods, particularly in underserved communities.
4. School and workplace programs: Implement school and workplace programs that promote the consumption of beta-glucan-rich foods, such as incorporating these foods into school meal programs or providing healthy snacks in the workplace.
5. Community outreach: Organize cooking classes, workshops, and seminars in local community centers to teach people how to incorporate beta-glucan-rich foods into their daily diets and share recipes highlighting these foods.
6. Healthcare professional training: Include information on the benefits of beta-glucans in the education and training of healthcare professionals, such as doctors,

nurses, and dietitians, to ensure they can provide evidence-based advice to their patients.

7. Research dissemination: Disseminate research findings on beta-glucans to the public through accessible channels, such as social media, public lectures, and webinars, to keep the public informed of the latest scientific developments.
8. Policy development: Advocate for the inclusion of beta-glucan-rich foods in dietary guidelines and public health policies, emphasizing their importance in the prevention and management of obesity, metabolic disorders, and other health conditions.
9. Public-private partnerships: Collaborate with food manufacturers to develop and promote healthier food products that are fortified with beta-glucans, ensuring they meet specific nutritional guidelines.
10. Monitoring and evaluation: Regularly monitor and evaluate the impact of public health initiatives emphasizing beta-glucans to ensure they are effective in improving public health outcomes and adjust strategies as needed.

By focusing on these future directions, public health initiatives can effectively promote the consumption of beta-glucan-rich foods and contribute to improving the overall health of communities.

REFERENCES

1. de Morais Junior AC, Schincaglia RM, Viana RB, Armet AM, Prado CM, Walter J, Mota JF (2023), The separate effects of whole oats and isolated beta-glucan on lipid profile: A systematic review and meta-analysis of randomized controlled trials. Clin Nutr ESPEN 53:224-237.
2. Du B, Bian Z, Xu B (2014), Skin health promotion effects of natural beta-glucan derived from cereals and microorganisms: a review. Phytother Res 28:159-166.
3. Du B, Meenu M, Liu H, Xu B (2019), A Concise Review on the Molecular Structure and Function Relationship of beta-Glucan. Int J Mol Sci 20.
4. Fernandez-Julia PJ, Munoz-Munoz J, van Sinderen D (2021), A comprehensive review on the impact of beta-glucan metabolism by Bacteroides and Bifidobacterium species as members of the gut microbiota. Int J Biol Macromol 181:877-889.
5. Ho HV, Sievenpiper JL, Zurbau A, Blanco Mejia S, Jovanovski E, Au-Yeung F, Jenkins AL, Vuksan V (2016), The effect of oat beta-glucan on LDL-cholesterol, non-HDL-cholesterol and apoB for CVD risk reduction: a systematic review and meta-analysis of randomised-controlled trials. Br J Nutr 116:1369-1382.
6. Ho HV, Sievenpiper JL, Zurbau A, Blanco Mejia S, Jovanovski E, Au-Yeung F, Jenkins AL, Vuksan V (2016), A systematic review and meta-analysis of randomized controlled trials of the effect of barley beta-glucan on LDL-C, non-HDL-C and apoB for cardiovascular disease risk reduction(i-iv). Eur J Clin Nutr 70:1239-1245.

7. Ikewaki N, Dedeepiya VD, Raghavan K, Rao KS, Vaddi S, Osawa H, Kisaka T, Kurosawa G, et al. (2022), beta-glucan vaccine adjuvant approach for cancer treatment through immune enhancement (B-VACCIEN) in specific immunocompromised populations (Review). Oncol Rep 47.
8. Liu Y, Wu Q, Wu X, Algharib SA, Gong F, Hu J, Luo W, Zhou M, et al. (2021), Structure, preparation, modification, and bioactivities of beta-glucan and mannan from yeast cell wall: A review. Int J Biol Macromol 173:445-456.
9. Maheshwari G, Sowrirajan S, Joseph B (2017), Extraction and Isolation of beta-Glucan from Grain Sources-A Review. J Food Sci 82:1535-1545.
10. Mallakpour S, Azadi E, Hussain CM (2021), Chitosan, alginate, hyaluronic acid, gums, and beta-glucan as potent adjuvants and vaccine delivery systems for viral threats including SARS-CoV-2: A review. Int J Biol Macromol 182:1931-1940.
11. Markovina N, Banjari I, Bucevic Popovic V, Jelicic Kadic A, Puljak L (2020), Efficacy and safety of oral and inhalation commercial beta-glucan products: Systematic review of randomized controlled trials. Clin Nutr 39:40-48.
12. Mathews R, Kamil A, Chu Y (2020), Global review of heart health claims for oat beta-glucan products. Nutr Rev 78:78-97.
13. Mathews R, Shete V, Chu Y (2021), The effect of cereal Beta-glucan on body weight and adiposity: A review of efficacy and mechanism of action. Crit Rev Food Sci Nutr:1-13.
14. Meena DK, Das P, Kumar S, Mandal SC, Prusty AK, Singh SK, Akhtar MS, Behera BK, et al. (2013), Beta-glucan: an ideal immunostimulant in aquaculture (a review). Fish Physiol Biochem 39:431-457.

15. Mejia SMV, de Francisco A, Bohrer B (2020), A comprehensive review on cereal beta-glucan: extraction, characterization, causes of degradation, and food application. Crit Rev Food Sci Nutr 60:3693-3704.
16. Mykhalevych A, Polishchuk G, Nassar K, Osmak T, Buniowska-Olejnik M (2022), beta-Glucan as a Techno-Functional Ingredient in Dairy and Milk-Based Products-A Review. Molecules 27.
17. Noronha JC, Zurbau A, Wolever TMS (2022), The importance of molecular weight in determining the minimum dose of oat beta-glucan required to reduce the glycaemic response in healthy subjects without diabetes: a systematic review and meta-regression analysis. Eur J Clin Nutr.
18. Yu J, Xia J, Yang C, Pan D, Xu D, Sun G, Xia H (2022), Effects of Oat Beta-Glucan Intake on Lipid Profiles in Hypercholesterolemic Adults: A Systematic Review and Meta-Analysis of Randomized Controlled Trials. Nutrients 14.
19. Zou Y, Liao D, Huang H, Li T, Chi H (2015), A systematic review and meta-analysis of beta-glucan consumption on glycemic control in hypercholesterolemic individuals. Int J Food Sci Nutr 66:355-362.
20. Zurbau A, Noronha JC, Khan TA, Sievenpiper JL, Wolever TMS (2021), The effect of oat beta-glucan on postprandial blood glucose and insulin responses: a systematic review and meta-analysis. Eur J Clin Nutr 75:1540-1554.
21. Pal, S., et al., 2011. The effect of a fibre supplement compared to a healthy diet on body composition, lipids, glucose, insulin and other metabolic syndrome risk factors in overweight and obese individuals. Br J Nutr. 105, 90-100.

Made in the USA
Monee, IL
08 November 2026

67994717R00083